THE
BACK
PAIN
RELIEF
DIET

DR. TODD SINETT

THE
BACK
PAIN
RELIEF
DIET

THE UNDISCOVERED KEY TO
REDUCING INFLAMMATION AND
ELIMINATING PAIN

Published by

EAST END PRESS

Bridgehampton, NY

ISBN: 978-0-9975304-7-6

Ebook ISBN: 978-0-9975304-8-3

Library of Congress Control Number: 2018909166

FIRST EDITION

Book Design by Pauline Neuwirth, Neuwirth & Associates

Cover Design by Tim Green

Manufactured in the United States of America

10 9 8 7 6 5 4 3 2 1

This book is dedicated to my beloved father, who had the determination to seek out a cure for his back pain and then the courage to share the undiscovered key with the world!

CONTENTS

──────── **PART III** ────────

MAINTAINING YOUR BACK-DIET CONNECTION
187

THE
BACK
PAIN
RELIEF
DIET

A PROBLEM WITH A NUTRITIONAL SOLUTION

Thank you for picking up *The Back Pain Relief Diet*. I am thanking you because I know a back pain relief diet book sounds a bit crazy, and there surely will be some people who won't open it for that reason. No doctor has ever discussed this in a dedicated text. In fact, most doctors who spend their lives treating back pain don't even know the link between diet and back pain. There are no diagnoses called "Inflamed Dietary Back Pain" or something referred to as DDD ("Degenerative Dietary Disease"), nor are there any high-tech diagnostic tests to help those who aren't looking beyond the back to identify diet as a source of inflammation and pain.

Suffice to say, I didn't invent this theory. However, we are in a worldwide back pain epidemic. Twenty percent of the population is currently suffering from back pain, and 85 percent will suffer from it at some point in their lives. Here are some other shocking truths about the back pain epidemic:

- In April 2014, back pain became the number one reason for job disability in the world.
- Back pain is second only to the common cold as the reason for visits to the doctor.
- Back pain is the third most common reason for hospitalization.
- It is the fifth most common reason for surgery.
- Thirty-three percent of all people over the age of 18 have sought treatment for back pain in the last five years.
- Our healthcare system spends upwards of $90 *billion* on the diagnosis and treatment of back pain.

All of these things show that our doctors are not succeeding in diagnosing and treating back pain, and that's because our treatments are not targeting all of the *sources* of back pain. Here's one more shocking truth about back pain: ones' diet continues to grow as a leading cause of back pain. This is one major contributing factor that your doctor is missing in diagnosing the source of your back problem.

It is not just that we are a nation of unhealthy eaters. Healthy eaters suffer from nutritionally induced back pain, too. That's why this book can help everyone identify their triggers. Yours may be sugar, or it may be kale! Yes, that super-food that can do no wrong *can* actually cause inflammation in the stomach and reflex into the back. The saying "We are what we eat" is a bit oversimplified. I would say, "We are what we digest." When your digestive system is upset, it creates gut inflammation, which ultimately causes muscular inflammation, resulting in pain.

Simply put: **Your diet could be the cause of your back pain. Conversely, your diet can also be the solution to your back pain.**

I will delve into the medicine behind the theory in more detail later, but here is the basic premise: all the parts of the body are interconnected. Anything that upsets your stomach causes inflammation. Consuming a large quantity of inflammatory foods causes your muscles to contract without relaxing. If this goes on for a prolonged period of time, back spasms and other negative health issues will result. Because your back and spine are closest to your stomach, the back is often the location where muscular pain and spasms stemming from stomach irritation first emerge. However, because your back and spine impact and connect to every part of your body, your pain may not actually be in your back. Instead, it may be emerging from elsewhere: your neck, feet, hips, really anywhere! There is no limit to the positive changes in your health when you reduce your chemical inflammation and when your digestive system improves in function.

How did I arrive at this theory? Well, it was actually my father's own health that led him to these conclusions decades ago and caused us both to refine our medical practices and develop the best way to analyze chemical and nutritional roots of back pain. Here is his story.

THE BACK PAIN PROBLEMS OF DR. SHELDON SINETT

For fifteen years, my father had been working from eight in the morning until eight at night as a chiropractor, seeing patient after patient, until one day, he bent down to pick up a tennis ball and could not get up. "I threw my back out," he said and took a few days off from work to rest in bed. However, the days turned into weeks, and the weeks turned into nine long months without any relief from his spasms and pain.

For those nine months, my father searched for answers to his back problem. My mother would drive him for doctor visits while my father lay down in the back of the car. He went for endless treatments and consultations within every known profession, including his own, but unfortunately, nothing helped. A surgeon recommended exploratory surgery (never a good term), offering to open him up to see if they could find anything. My father and family were desperate to find an answer to his suffering. Hoping to find another option, he went to see a doctor in Detroit with the fortuitous name of Dr. George Goodheart. Dr. Goodheart was unlike any other doctor that my father had seen. He focused solely on one question: *why* was my father having such terrible back spasms? He reasoned that other doctors were focusing on getting rid of the back spasms rather than finding out why they occurred in the first place. Dr. Goodheart told my father that back pain always comes from somewhere or something: the only thing that is random in the body is trauma, such as a car accident or falling off of a bike; otherwise, back pain builds little by little. Eventually, a simple movement, such as bending down, can become the proverbial straw that broke the camel's back. The doctor told my father that while we may not always understand the cause, it is likely that something is being missed by the doctors, preventing them from diagnosing the problem. Dr. Goodheart surmised that, other than his back pain, my father seemed to be in good physical condition, that his back pain certainly didn't come about from some trauma or accident, and that bending down to pick up that tennis ball wasn't the true cause of his agony. Dr. Goodheart then looked to my father's diet, which included quite a lot of caffeine and sugar. The good doctor felt that was the missing piece.

I can assure you that no one was more disbelieving than my father. The simple reason was that my father had made his living helping people who were suffering from back pain, and nowhere in his training or studies did he ever hear about diet (diet, of all things!) causing back pain.

But after all traditional and non-traditional treatments failed to bring my father some relief, he was left with two options: to change his diet or to have the exploratory surgery. He chose to change his diet, reasoning that if option one didn't work, he could always opt for surgery. Dr. Goodheart treated him just a few times in conjunction with a complete change in his nutrition, and, lo and behold, my father was cured in just a few short weeks. Within about a month he was back on the tennis court. He kept up with his new lifestyle, and he never suffered from back pain for the rest of his life.

After getting his "life" back, my father returned to his practice with a very different perspective and approach. Because of his own back pain experience (a problem that had been solved with a change in nutrition), he examined and treated patients quite differently, and he achieved astounding results. Soon, he was sought after by many of the world's rich and famous in their pursuit of ridding themselves of back pain. I joined my father in practice in 1995 and had the pleasure of practicing with him for about ten years.

MY OWN AHA MOMENT

While my own "aha" dietary back pain moment was not as dramatic as my father's, it was pretty profound. As a New Year's resolution, I decided to go on a real health kick. Even though I don't drink alcohol or coffee or indulge in a lot of sweets, I wanted to improve my diet: no more sweets or simple carbohydrates for me! I decided I was going to have high-fiber oatmeal every day for breakfast, a salad for lunch, and lean proteins for dinner. After a week into this diet, I was hoping to notice a difference in my energy levels and overall well-being. The changes that I experienced were mind-blowing to me. Yes, my energy levels changed—as did my sense of well-being; however, both got *significantly worse*. I asked myself, How was this possible? I had a dramatic increase in bloating and stomach pain, and eventually I suffered a stiff neck, which seemed to worsen by the day. My neck, shoulders, and upper back got so tight I could barely turn my head or bend. There were no changes in my exercise; I didn't sleep funny nor were there any changes in my routine other than my eating habits. What had happened? Could it actually be possible that the change in my diet was the cause of my muscular pain? I immediately returned to my old eating habits, which had been pretty healthy, and within two days, I felt significantly better.

What I learned from my own experience led me to a whole new understanding of nutrition. It also answered a question that had alluded me for years. How was it that patients who were eating healthy diets still seemed to be suffering from dietary/digestive back pain? Could it be that oatmeal or salads were less healthy than a bagel or a sandwich? For me, I would say the answer is yes. I understand that a bagel may be less nutritious compared to oatmeal; however, my body digested and functioned better when eating a bagel for breakfast than when eating oatmeal. My body seemingly reacted well to a turkey sandwich, but after eating salad, I would feel gassy and bloated, resulting in diarrhea.

There are many stories or proverbs that state that from difficult moments come great things or that great challenges result in great achievements. For my family, my father's severe, debilitating back pain was that difficult moment, and thankfully it turned out to be the biggest blessing, not only for him and my family, but I hope also for you. I trust this book will be your guide to understanding digestive-caused pain and to learning how to better feed your body. With a change in your nutrition, you will be able to repair your system and achieve greater physical health from head to toe.

THE SINETT SOLUTION

Who am I, and how am I qualified to write this book and help treat you from afar? Here's a little bit about my career using what I refer to as the Sinett Solution: this is the practice of listening to the signs from your whole body and treating all sources of pain on structural, digestive, and emotional levels to achieve what we call a triad of health.

For more than two decades, I have been practicing medicine at my wellness center, located on Madison Avenue in New York City. The unique approach and treatment style of my practice follows the philosophy that had helped my father back in 1975. I have put together a team of the finest doctors, all with different training and approaches, to try to get to the bottom of why a patient may be suffering. I say we specialize in personalized whole care.

In 2006, after research and repeated complaints from patients, I discovered a commonality among most back pain sufferers: discomfort brought on by the forward hunch that we are all developing due to hours of sitting in front of our computers, sitting in our cars, or bent over our smart phones. I realized the modern world was making us sick! Specifically, on a structural level, I realized that we all need more extension in our backs to reverse the effects of our daily routines on the spine. I created a back-pain-relieving product called the Backbridge, which is designed to decompress one's spine by gradually and safely realigning one's posture with one simple stretch. The continued gradual extension that the Backbridge provides allows a patient to undo all of that forward posture. My father and I wrote a book to explain our new findings about the triad of health and debunk untruths and misconceptions about back pain. In 2008, *Truth About Back Pain* was published just after my father's passing. To date, I have sold almost 40,000 Backbridges worldwide, and it is truly rewarding to receive emails of thanks from people all over the world, people whom I have never met but who have been helped by the Backbridge.

In 2015, I released my second back book to expand on and update the principles of my first book. *3 Weeks to a Better Back* allows readers who are back pain sufferers to self-diagnose and self-treat their back pain on three different levels: the structural, nutritional, and emotional. The nutritional component is explained in that book, which offers alternate recipes to those recipes and preparations found in this one.

I elaborated on structural treatments in my third book, *The Ultimate Backbridge Stretch Book.* While my Backbridge Extension Stretch was the key stretch that I offered patients in my office, many began to ask for new stretches. At about the same time, I noticed that yoga and Pilates instructors and fitness trainers were experimenting with additional uses of the Backbridge. With their help, I developed a detailed picture book that allows the reader to regain flexibility and good posture by using the Backbridge as an assist in a variety of different stretches for head-to-toe relief. (For more information or to purchase a backbridge, visit backbridge.com.)

THE TRIAD OF HEALTH

To summarize, my first three books delve into what is known as the triad of health: structure, nutrition, and emotion. Each element of the triage can cause significant back pain. Most people have areas of structural care, nutrition, and emotional care that they could improve. By making modifications to how we treat the body (structural care), what we eat (nutrition), and how we manage stress (emotional care), most of us will experience dramatically increased comfort in the back and other parts of the body. *The Back Pain Relief Diet*, while addressing only one part of the greater solution, is important—and deserving of its own title—because so many people do not make the connection between nutrition and back pain. Read on, and this book will help give you:

- an understanding of the medicine behind the back-diet connection
- stories of those patients who have been helped by my meal plans
- a Digestive Inflammation Test to help you determine if your back pain has a digestive cause
- a Diagnostic Nutrition Test to help you determine which foods are causing your digestive distress
- a choice of four different meal plans tailored to your sensitivities to reduce inflammation and heal your back
- a Symptom Journal to record your journey to health through a change in your nutrition.

I am downright excited to present this material to you because I know that there are thousands, if not millions, of people who can be helped with this information. It could be your missing piece and the difference between your getting to have a healthy active lifestyle or a life filled with "managing your back pain," which usually means a life filled with pain and pain medications. If, upon taking the tests that follow in Chapters 3 and 4, you find you are suffering from back pain because of your diet, the great news is that this is a problem with an easy and cheap solution and that you will feel better in just a few weeks. There are so many people who think they cannot change their ways when it comes to nutrition, and, as a doctor, there is nothing more rewarding than helping people find a nutritional balance and, as a result, feel good. So many emotions go into eating, and taking control of your diet and finding that middle ground of health and fun can really help improve the way you feel about yourself and your body. Happily, the nutrition treatment can dramatically impact and improve the other two areas on my triad of health.

MEAL PLANS FROM WILLOW JAROSH AND STEPHANIE CLARKE

Nutritionists Willow Jarosh and Stephanie Clarke help those of my patients who I believe are suffering from digestive-induced back pain. They contributed the meal plans that you will find in this book. They met in the combined Dietetic Internship and Master's program in Nutrition Communication at Tufts University's Friedman School of Nutrition Science and Policy and went on to cofound C&J Nutrition. Their philosophy is both simple and realistic: nutritional programs need to be sustainable and should focus on finding recipes that bring health and enjoyment together in order to ensure long-term success. Their recipes integrate some twists on old favorites while also addressing different types of digestive needs and surely will help those with a wide array of food sensitivities.

One Patient's Story

I HAD CHRONIC LOW-BACK issues forever—since I was eighteen years old. The pain was on and off, but mostly on, and I went through periods of debilitating, depressing pain. I remember trying to get out of bed on many occasions, lying on the floor in agony and having to crawl to the bathroom. I tried everything to get out of pain: from chiropractors to acupuncture to physical therapy and medication. I went to see a colleague of Dr. Sinett's in New Jersey, and we weren't making any progress. He said he had a great friend, who just wrote a book, and suggested my picking up a copy. He told me if it resonated with me, I should make an appointment with him. I bought the book—Dr. Sinett's first, *The Truth About Back Pain*. For the first time, I began to look at things more holistically. Instead of focusing in on my low back pain, I learned about the chemical and emotional issues that can affect how we feel. The doctors whom I had seen hadn't thought to address the underlying causes!

When I made an appointment with Dr. Sinett, his receptionist said I could bring my copy of *The Truth About Back Pain* with me, and that Dr. Sinett would be happy to sign it. After years of pain, I was still skeptical and told her I would let him autograph my book when he cured me!

On the day of the appointment, I arrived—without my copy of the book—and sat in the waiting room, which was fairly full. Dr. Sinett walked out of an exam room with a patient, came over to me with a big smile on his face, extended his hand, and told me it was a pleasure to meet me and that I wouldn't have to wait much longer. That made an impression. It isn't often that a New York City doctor in a busy practice takes the time to come out and say hello!

Dr. Sinett took my X-rays during that first appointment, and when I came back for the results, he put the scans on the board to reveal the frontal view of my spine. I thought it looked like I had massive amounts of stomach cancer, and I got nervous. I said, "What are those circles in my body?"

The answer was gas. Dr. Sinett told me I had a good deal of indigestion and turned his attention first to my diet. I didn't realize I had indigestion! We talked about my intake, and he recommended I keep a food diary and come back in two weeks with a picnic basket of my usual food to sample in the office. When I returned, I ate my picnic basket, and Dr. Sinett did a physical examination instead of blood work. He turned his attention to the repetition that I had noted in my food diary and the inflammation he was feeling after I consumed my lunch. I always ate a turkey sandwich on whole wheat bread, a bag of pretzels, and a can of diet soda. I admitted, after eating this lunch, I would always get bloated—to the point of having to let my belt out a notch. He suggested gluten and caffeine might be causing my pain. I had never heard of gluten at that point. I have always been pretty health conscious and thought whole wheat bread and pretzels instead of chips were the better options.

For the next ten days, I cut gluten and caffeine out of my diet. I immediately dropped seven pounds of bloat and felt awesome. My health improved very quickly; it wasn't gradual. I am in the hotel industry and travel frequently, and I no longer had to sit on bags of ice when I flew! I felt amazing, and I went from having trouble walking and sitting to running a 5K in just a few weeks. After running that 5K, I considered myself cured and brought my copy of *The Truth About Back Pain* in to Dr. Sinett to sign.

The catalyst for my recovery was the diet, and from there, we were able to look at the other factors that contributed to my pain. We realized that the arch of my foot wasn't optimal, and I began wearing custom-made orthotics. I began using the Backbridge several times a day to negate my C-posture. We also worked on dealing with my stress. The realization that stress can impact the way you feel was eye opening to me and helped me readjust my mental outlook. Stress from work would lock everything up in my spine and compound the issue.

Now, ten years later, I still use the Backbridge, manage my stress, and make sure that I keep variety in my diet. I still avoid gluten, soda, and sodium. The combination has kept me healthy for a decade after a young adulthood of pain.

Other than curing my back pain, one other thing has really stuck with me about Dr. Sinett. Upon leaving his office after that first appointment, he called me from his cell phone to tell me how great it was to meet me, reassured me he could help, and told me I was free to call him any time. In addition to being able to see the underlying causes of your pain, he's a really good guy—a caring guy who has become a good friend. It's a very special thing in a doctor.

—*Kevin Dailey*

I started off by thanking you for picking up this book, but my hope is that at the end of the book, you will be on the beginning of your journey to lifelong good health and will be able to thank yourself for taking this opportunity to try something new, something perhaps unconventional and a bit odd, and ultimately, finding relief from your pain. What do you have to lose, other than your back pain?

—*Dr. Todd Sinett*

PART I

CAUSES AND TREATMENT OF BACK PAIN

1.

INFLAMMATION AND THE CAUSES OF BACK PAIN

Before I elaborate on the causes of back pain, I would like readers to understand the ways in which the parts of the body are interconnected. Specifically, it's important to see just how inflammation affects the back.

Inflammation, or swelling, as well as redness and pain, are normally part of a healthy immune response. When an injury occurs, inflammation is initiated to help your body protect that injured part. The body also produces elevated levels of cortisol, a hormone that maintains the body's connective tissue and begins the healing process following an injury. However, when your cortisol levels have been elevated for a prolonged period of time, you develop chronic inflammation, which actually destroys healthy tissue and has been found to cause or be a factor in cancer, diabetes, depression, heart disease, stroke, and Alzheimer's disease. To this list of ailments, I would add back pain, as well as tension in the muscles, ligaments, tendons, and discs. It is chronic inflammation that makes our backs susceptible to "going out" after we make simple movements.

There are three causes of chronic inflammation resulting in back pain:

1. **Structural Inflammation.** This is the swelling found in muscles, bones, discs, nerves, and posture, and it is the most obvious and easy-to-understand culprit. During the day, our bodies undergo an almost endless list of physical stressors—whether it be from lugging bags, commuting, sitting all day in uncomfortable chairs in an office, walking in unsupportive footwear. All of these things cause irritation and inflammation. Those in the medical field currently spend the large majority of their resources on diagnosing and treating back pain for structural causes alone. Unfortunately, based on back pain statistics, the treatment results are quite unsuccessful, proving that our laser-focus on just structural inflammation is an incomplete approach to treatment.

2. **Emotional Inflammation.** In a landmark study, researchers at Stanford University discovered that stress combined with emotional outlook was the number one factor for back pain. When our bodies are under prolonged periods of stress, our levels of cortisol, known as our stress hormone, spike, triggering the inflammatory response and causing our mind and back to become uptight. Our society has ever so slowly acknowledged the role our emotional tension is having on our backs. Therapeutic practices such as mindfulness and meditation are becoming more and more commonplace, and therapy is viewed as a helpful treatment for back pain.

3. **Nutritional or Digestive Inflammation.** This area is most lacking in medical research. It is also the area least understood or acknowledged by back pain sufferers—and is consequently the impetus for *The Back Pain Relief Diet*. The remainder of this chapter will deal specifically with nurturing a better understanding of the role of digestive inflammation in our daily lives and the extent to which it can harm your body.

THE DEAL WITH DIGESTION

The world of digestive upsets is not a welcoming one. You may be aware that you have a sensitive stomach, but you may not realize how far-reaching the chemical effects are on the rest of your body.

Our bodies react to what we eat or drink with a viscerosomatic response. *Viscero* means "organ"; *somatic* refers to the body—in this case, the musculoskeletal system. Some of what we consume is soothing to the body; some irritates it and causes pain. This viscerosomatic response to what we eat can range from being alert after morning coffee, to feeling sleepy from the tryptophan in turkey, to getting an upset stomach from something acidic, to developing back pain. Have you ever been hung over? You probably remember the headache, as well as the upset stomach. But try to recall: *how did your muscles feel?* Loose and limber or tight and achy? You probably didn't feel like exercising nor would you have a good workout if you tried. This was a viscerosomatic reaction to alcohol and is an example of what happens to your body over time with foods that create inflammation. Because there isn't usually an immediate reaction to the wrong foods unless you have a food allergy—such as lactose intolerance, for instance—the connection isn't often made. In fact, the most overlooked cause of back pain is diet. While there are thousands of studies on how nutrition impacts muscular function, very few health professionals have connected the dots between digestive function and nutrition to back pain. Chronic pain, particularly in the back, can be tied to body inflammation. This is not the kind of inflammation or swelling you see with an acute injury, but instead chronic inflammation can occur internally throughout the body in response to a poor diet that results in low digestive function.

POOR DIETS AND OTHER PROBLEMS

Studies confirm that there is an association between back pain and being overweight or obese. The correlation seems obvious: the more you weigh, the more your bones—especially the spine—must bear. Interestingly, some studies also suggest that the association may not be only musculoskeletal, but that obesity-related stomach inflammation caused by the toxicity of unhealthy eating may also play a role in low back pain. Therefore, recommendations for a healthful diet to help treat back pain for anyone who is overweight or obese are warranted.

In a 1995 report published in *The Lancet*, researchers in Finland corroborated this perspective when they conducted autopsies on people who died from non-related back issues but who were on record as having suffered from back pain. What they discovered was that people who had suffered from back pain had many more blocked arteries to the spine than people who never had back pain troubles. This was proof that poor diet choices can and do clog arteries!

In another study published in the *Asian Spine Journal* in 2014, researchers reported that 31 percent of women and 24.6 percent of men who were suffering from back pain also suffered from gastrointestinal (GI) complaints such as abdominal pain or food intolerance. I see a similar percentage of patients who have both GI complaints and stomach inflammation, as well as back or other muscular pain. When these patients tell me that they are frustrated with their body and feel like they can hardly live, much less work out optimally, I point out the choices of Olympic athletes as a good model. Olympians are extremely particular in their diets because they believe that the right nutrition will make them stronger. The reverse is also true: the wrong diet will weaken their muscular system function or cause back and other muscular pain. Other poor eating habits—such as stuffing yourself with large meals, skipping meals, or consuming only low-carb foods—can result in low blood sugar and create more stress in the body. All of these factors can ultimately trigger an inflammatory reaction in the stomach which results in back pain.

In my practice, I've seen many cases of people complaining of back pain, but this is especially true from patients who say they don't have much time to prepare meals. Typically, I ask them to keep a daily food log; the average log looks something like this:

Breakfast: coffee, muffin or bagel, more coffee
Lunch: sandwich, chips, soda or iced tea
Snack: candy or chips, soda or coffee
Dinner: pizza or pasta, soda or wine, pastry or ice cream

Your body is a high-performance engine, and filling it with low-performance fuels doesn't provide nearly enough of the vitamins and nutrients you need to function. The choices listed above will not only result in energy crashes, but they also will irritate the delicate balance of your digestive system, creating inflammation.

On the flip side, about 20 percent of patients I encounter describe themselves as "health nuts." Fruits and vegetables—including big raw salads, smoothies, and other roughage—are the foundation of their diets. They also suffer from back pain induced by digestive issues. These people are eating too much of a good thing, and the lack of variety in their diets as well as the over-consumption of one or two food groups irritates their digestive systems. These patients complain of gassiness, bloating, abdominal pain, diarrhea, and even constipation. Ultimately, we need multiple sources of vitamins, minerals, and other nutrients, and when it comes to the right diet for the body, balance and variety are key. By introducing whole grains, more protein and even some dairy, the transit time becomes more accommodating for positive absorption, and stomach inflammation and its related back pain goes away.

A DEEPER LOOK AT THE CONNECTIONS BETWEEN DIET, EMOTION, AND STRUCTURE

So now you know that there are three causes of back pain: structural causes, dietary causes, and emotional causes. It is really important to recognize how interlinked these three causes are. While your pain may be primarily driven by dietary issues, it's important to understand how an issue may be compounded by other causes.

THE DIGESTIVE AND EMOTIONAL LINK

The link between emotions and eating has been well publicized, but, in my opinion, is misunderstood. The connection goes much deeper than "emotional eating." Your emotional state when consuming a meal or a snack dramatically determines your digestive process.

Here's an example: if you are eating a hot fudge sundae when you are depressed, there is a completely different biochemical process than if you are having the sundae as part of a celebration. Your body produces different neuro-peptides and hormones in a state of depression than it does in a state of happiness, and this affects how your metabolism functions. It also explains why people could go wildly off their normally regimented diet on vacation and feel great; however, if they did that in their normal environment, they would suffer terribly. This also explains how one person might eat very little and not lose weight, while another person might take in more calories and seem not to gain weight.

Stress and emotions are causes of back and stomach pain in their own right. Just think about the havoc that can be wreaked when stress is paired with an onslaught of digestive irritants. I experienced this firsthand. Right after my father passed away, I had a lot of stomach pain after drinking orange juice. When I was in a state of acute grief, I just couldn't digest all that acid. It wasn't until a year later that I could finally drink orange juice in the morning without it bothering me. This is where mindful, or intuitive, eating, which we'll learn more about in Chapter 2, comes significantly into play. Ask yourself, "Am I eating with regret or joy?" "Am I feeling differently after consuming certain foods during times of stress?" Simply put, a healthy relationship with eating is vital to being healthy, and awareness of the strong correlation between stomach and stress is essential to achieving that goal.

THE STRUCTURAL AND DIGESTIVE CONNECTION

The structural relationship to digestive function is very much overlooked but, in my opinion, is indisputable. A common example of a structural treatment affecting digestive function is the Heimlich maneuver. When performing the Heimlich when someone is choking, you are literally able to manually impact the digestive function—or, in this case, the non-digestive function.

A less examined structural factor on digestion is your posture. If you slouch most of the day, your posture actually impedes your digestive process by decreasing the space between your chest and stomach. Proper posture can actually help you digest your food more optimally. So, heed your mom's advice, and don't slouch at the dinner table!

Another overlooked structural impact on digestive function is visceral manipulations (commonly known as massage or manual treatments). While your small intestine digests food, your large intestine excretes food or eliminates the waste material. The ileocecal valve is a sphincter muscle valve that separates the small and large intestine and prevents the waste material from returning into the small intestine. This valve is under nerve control so it is affected by digestive secretions and diet function as well as by stress. If the valve isn't working properly, toxins that should be exiting your body will essentially back up into your small intestine, create excess gas, and cause back pain. You can correct this valve's function by pushing your hands in your gut between your belly button and right hip, angling the pressure towards your left shoulder. Hold the pressure for approximately thirty seconds to a minute. This will frequently be a bit sensitive. You can also ice this point for fifteen minutes every hour. As you continue to improve, this point will decrease in sensitivity. I often perform this maneuver on my patients, and while they don't like it, it does help!

My patient Kristen is a great example of someone whose digestive upsets greatly aggravated a structural problem. For her, although diet wasn't a cure, it did provide tremendous reduction in her overall pain.

One Patient's Story

ABOUT TWO YEARS AGO, I herniated a disc. I experienced pain throughout my low back which radiated down my left side, into the glute and piriformis. I was working at a physical therapy office at the time, and, following the herniation, I did four months of physical therapy, chiropractic care, and active release therapy. After receiving an epidural, I met a friend who recommended Dr. Sinett.

When I finally made an appointment with Dr. Sinett about six months ago, I realized he was a chiropractor. I assumed he was just going to do adjustments, which I had already received. But to my surprise, on my first visit, he began with kinesiology tests and pressed on various points of my abdomen. I was in so much pain—practically on the verge of tears!

Dr. Sinett knew right away what the problem was! He told me I had a lot of inflammation and that he had a diet for me. He even told me that pain from stomach inflammation can mask itself as a herniated disk. We took a look at my diet, but I am a foodie, and my diet was full of everything! It was hard to tell what I was sensitive to. So, he recommended I start with a strict Elimination Diet to cleanse my system and then gradually reintroduce foods to see what caused pain.

When I started the diet, I immediately felt lighter and better. Within a week, my skin got better, I wasn't puffy or bloated, and the radiating pain down my back and into the hip reduced to one specific spot in the back (which did turn out to be a herniated disc). But the diet made clearer where the actual physical pain was coming from.

Ultimately, it turned out I was sensitive to dairy and eggs. Prior to meeting Dr. Sinett, I was eating eggs every day, along with Ezekiel bread with grass-fed butter and coffee with half-and-half. I had been a personal trainer in the nineties and until my back injury, I liked to exercise and ate everything I wanted. I felt like if it was good quality and organic, it was healthy for me. I especially thought that eggs were healthy. I didn't understand my system and body. I thought I felt good and didn't even realize how inflamed I was until he did that abdomen test!

Ever since, I've kept dairy and eggs out of my diet. I've only tried eggs twice, and one time in particular, I had major stomach pains and got sick. I was able to add back everything else to my diet and still feel good. Occasionally, during the holidays and parties, I indulge, but I always wind up sick. Now I'm very aware of my sensitivities, and that helps me make choices that are good for me.

I didn't get totally healed (I still had the herniated disc), but Dr. Sinett helped me understand the concept that certain healthy foods may not be healthy for me, and changing my nutrition greatly improved my health and overall pain.

—Kristen Sofia

2.

THE 10 BASIC PRINCIPLES OF THE BACK-DIET CONNECTION

Your lifestyle should be about finding what's right for your body, both nutritionally and digestively. These ten principles will help you listen to your body and find out what it needs.

Principle 1.

Regardless of your type of diet, your diet can be the cause of your back pain.

Whether you eat a "healthy" diet or an "unhealthy" diet, whether you are "vegan" or eat "paleo," whether you start your day with a green drink or an 18-ounce cup of coffee, whether you eat pizza or salad for lunch, your back pain may be stemming from your diet. As I learned from my own "Aha moment" (described in my Introduction), a diet needs to be healthy for YOU and YOUR DIGESTIVE SYSTEM, and everyone's intestines are a little bit different. This means that what someone else deems "healthy" may not be right for you.

Principle 2.

Regardless of your symptoms, diagnosis, or the severity of your back pain, your diet may be the cause of your pain.

It doesn't matter if you suffer from a nagging tight back or the kind of severe back pain that is incapacitating. Even if you have been diagnosed with a herniated disc, sciatica, degenerative disc disease, or spinal stenosis, your diet could still be the cause of much of your suffering. Because more than 99 percent of doctors, probably including your doctors, haven't explored the link between diet and back pain, they likely didn't have this knowledge when crafting your diagnosis. I will disparage my profession in a sense when I say that because most doctors feel such responsibility to give a diagnosis, even when they don't know the cause, they will diagnose back pain and attribute it to a structural cause. Even if your diagnosis came from a diagnostic test, it may not be fully accurate. The only test that can help identify a root cause of digestive inflammation is an endoscopy, or a doctor who is trained to detect gut inflammation by applying pressure to various points on the abdomen.

THE MRI MYTH

Lots of doctors—and thus their patients—still believe that an MRI, or magnetic resonance imaging, is helpful in diagnosing back pain. In fact, this testing is so common that many of my patients come in and demand that I send them for an MRI. The thinking is that a disc or bone is pressing on a nerve root and that the MRI study can be used to observe what is happening to that nerve. Stanley J. Bigos, professor emeritus of Orthopedic Surgery and Environmental Health at the University of Washington in Seattle, explained the appeal of the MRI when he said, "The reality is patients want an answer, the doctor wants to get the patient out of the room and the hypotheses start to flow."

For some reason, studies that refute the power of the MRI have not resonated. For example, researchers of a study published in the *New England Journal of Medicine* in 1994 reported that MRIs were conducted on ninety-eight people who were *symptom-free* of back pain. Sixty-four percent of these people showed clear evidence of a bulging or protruding disc and 28 percent showed disc herniation—spinal abnormalities that would seem to indicate severe back ailments. However, because these people did not complain of back pain, the idea of diagnosing pain solely from an MRI is misguided.

Doctors at the University of Washington then concluded in 1998 and 2000 that MRIs resulted in a higher rate of specialist consultations and more surgeries but *fewer* beneficial outcomes. In 2003, in the June issue of the *Journal of the American Medical Association,* the authors detailed a controlled randomized trial that proved that X-rays were better than MRIs for diagnosing issues of lower back pain and in fact led to fewer patient interventions and ultimately fewer surgeries.

Why then don't MRIs produce better outcomes for back pain sufferers? The reason is that MRIs do not take the root cause of the pain into account. They serve only to bolster the notion that back pain is nothing more than the symptom of an underlying disease. Many conventional physicians and surgeons miss the true causes of back pain, because they continue to be stuck on the easy explanation offered by high-tech imaging. All too often, the orthopedist who sees a herniated disc on an MRI decides that the only answer is surgery. They don't consider nutritional and emotional elements that could ease the added stress to the physical abnormality and provide natural relief. In cases where no structural abnormality is found, patients are typically sent off with a prescription for anti-inflammatory drugs or other painkillers. Painkillers are not real solutions. They are not a cure. They merely mask the pain.

Because you now understand that all parts of the body are interconnected, you can see how finding and fixing just a localized issue means that both the doctor and the patient are missing the bigger picture—including lots of potential causes of your pain. If your back pain is caused by a foot imbalance radiating up the body and into the spine, an MRI of the back will not reveal the problem in your foot. If your back pain is caused by emotional stress or a digestive upset, an MRI won't tell you this either! Localized issues can be improved—without surgery—by fixing the true cause!

Ultimately, "true but unrelated" sums up MRI findings. An MRI may find structural irregularities, causing the doctor to attempt to connect your symptoms to those irregularities. This model has proven not to work. My model, which takes into account all of the possible sources of global pain, will tell you so much more about your body and why you are suffering than an MRI ever could. And with that core information can come an effective (and less invasive) solution—the Sinett Solution!

Principle 3.

Before undergoing any kind of invasive back procedure, rule out diet as your cause!

The most important creed that doctors are taught is a Latin phrase "premium nil nocere," which means "first do no harm." The information and premise of this book certainly aligns with this saying, but our current aggressive structural treatments are violating this principle. The failure rate for back surgeries is so prevalent that it has its own diagnosis, called Failed Back Surgical Syndrome (FBSS). Barring a spinal medical emergency, the treatment of back pain rarely requires immediate action. Invasive back treatments, such as surgery, can come with some serious medical risks and complications. You don't want to take on those risks unnecessarily if the solution may be as simple as changing what you eat and drink. Before publication of this book, diet-induced back pain wasn't even considered an option, an oversight that has resulted in many unnecessary and failed surgical treatments. Take your time to rule out diet as a cause. For example, my patient Jon did not do this until after a surgery failed to cure him; ultimately, he discovered nutrition to be the key to restoring his back and his life.

One Patient's Story

I HAVE SOMETHING CALLED degenerative disc disease and have had a poor back for the best part of ten years. The key thing about my condition is that the problem is at many levels (T9 through L4), not just in one segment of the back. In 2010, I had a major surgery in London, where I lived at the time, which resulted in the insertion of two titanium rods and 14 screws from T9 through L4, as well as the fusion of a couple of vertebrae from T11 to L1. After struggling with the metal, I had the surgery reversed and the rods and screws removed in 2012.

Around that time, I moved to the United States for work and discovered Dr. Sinett. He sat me down and spoke about his unique approach. Dr. Sinett then did some very strange maneuvers in his office, lifting my arms and legs and such. He talked about structural care but specifically honed in on my diet. I'm in okay shape, I exercise, and I didn't think I ate too poorly. But he wanted more than that. He rubbed my gut and told me that my stomach was inflamed and irritated. I had no idea it was irritated! He then talked about toxicity and his diet for back pain. I told my friends and they thought it was strange, because some of the things I was permitted to eat on the diet, like nuts, were high in calories! Dr. Sinett's diet had a totally different approach. It was not a weight loss diet, but a diet to reduce my gut inflammation. Nuts, as he explained, are low in toxins, so they were on his "Yes" list.

It took me six months to buy into Dr. Sinett's nutrition plan. For that time, I'd do the diet for three days, then the weekend came, and I'd forget it. It was so unique to anything I had seen or witnessed, I just wasn't convinced—and after living in London and Dubai, I had seen a whole host of doctors and experienced many different facets of international healthcare! But with Dr. Sinett, you can't cheat, because if you go in there for a few weeks and say you have been doing the diet, he can just feel your gut and other points on your body and tell pretty quickly that you haven't! Ultimately, I was kidding myself.

Finally, I committed to the diet for a month, which led to two months, because I noticed marked improvement in my pain. On his diet, you don't go hungry! You can eat plenty of food and it isn't complex to follow; there is just a list of things to avoid. Even though the diet isn't calorie controlled, after a few months, I surprisingly lost twenty-four pounds. I felt a lot better because I wasn't bloated or sore. I wasn't even aware I was bloated or sore until it wasn't even there! I learned that if your gut is upset, pain can radiate around to your back. So the diet is massive, and for me, it's been very helpful when it seemed little else was helping.

Now, I follow Dr. Sinett's diet, I work to keep my emotions in check, and I meet with the physical therapist in his office to keep myself in structural health, which is complementary, and there aren't many facilities that I've found that offer that set-up. If I go out of sync on one of those three things, I fall down. I've just had a great Christmas, for example, but a rubbish Christmas from my diet perspective, and I know I have to knuckle back on it, because I have the confidence now that getting on track will keep my back up to par. I can manage my process a lot better having met Dr. Sinett.

From a surgical perspective, my major operation was technically perfect. It just didn't help me. Dr. Sinett could have helped without my having had the surgery at all, and anyone with back pain facing surgery should certainly see Dr. Sinett as a matter of course.

—Jon Mann

Principle 4.

You will know your answer in less than a month, and for a lot of people, within just two weeks!

The Diagnostic Nutrition Test in Chapter 4 will help you figure out your potential food allergens and create a tailored diet. Your body will respond quickly. If food is indeed a primary cause of your pain, then you will feel a significant difference after following the nutrition plan for just a few weeks. If not, then you will know to turn your attention to structural or emotional issues. My book *3 Weeks to a Better Back* deals with solutions to these causes as well.

Principle 5.

The cause of most back pain isn't just one factor.

Most back pain isn't just one factor but rather a compilation of issues: posture, stress, weight, job, activity levels—the list goes on. However, diet is a huge missing piece that we all should take a look at. Maybe your diet change will translate into a one hundred percent improvement in your back pain; maybe it will be 33 percent (stress and/or structure being the other 66 percent of the cause). Regardless, it should improve your quality of life and help you achieve a total cure in conjunction with other treatments to achieve the health triad.

Principle 6.

Just because a particular food is healthy or nutritious doesn't mean it is healthy for you!

I always felt diets were so confusing. How can one author be touting the benefits of a vegan diet while another touts the benefits of a paleo diet? How can one diet be high protein and low carb, and the other be low protein and high carb? Which diet is right and which diet is wrong? The answer is that they are both right and both wrong. The real question, which was the moral of my "Aha moment," is, "What is right for you?" Some people function better eating more proteins while others function better having more carbohydrates. Once you find out which diet or foods are uniquely right for you, you can rid yourself of your excess gas and your diet-induced back pain. The digestive solutions in Part

II ("Proper Foods and Practical Meal Plans") will help you figure out which diet is right for you and which isn't ideal.

Principle 7.

The quality of your bowel movements determines the quality of your digestive system, which determines the health of your back.

When talking about diet, we seem concerned only with what a person is eating (input), but we also need to look carefully at the output to understand fully how the body is digesting and excreting the foods. Our bodies and back will not only function as well as the fuel we put into it (input) but also as well as how we eliminate our waste material (output).

THE SCOOP ON POOP

Before we identify your specific nutrition sensitivities, let's address output and how you are currently completing the digestive process. The quality of your output directly correlates to how your nutrients affect you and therefore to the health of your back!

One of the most common but missed causes of back pain is improper bowel movements, that is, constipation and diarrhea. When a person is regularly constipated, the body builds up waste material that should be exiting the body in a timely manner but instead winds up not exiting when necessary. This increasing internal toxicity impacts your muscular system by elevating the inflammatory factor. Diarrhea can result in the same type of inflammatory reaction from the body; however, with diarrhea, the intestinal system is unable to properly process the waste material and excretes it too soon, irritating the intestinal system. An irritated digestive and intestinal system can then affect the muscular system. In short, what you put in must be processed effectively by your digestive system and excreted in a healthy, consistent way.

Normal bowel habits do vary. When we talk about regularity, what we're really talking about is *what's regular for you.* Three

Bristol Stool Chart

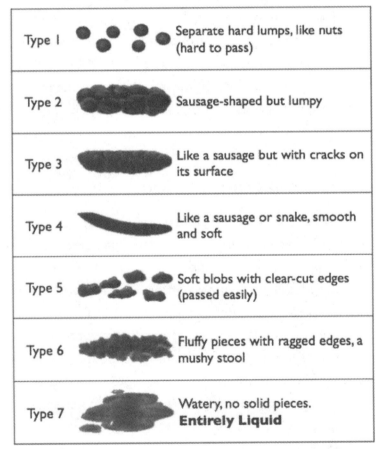

Type 1		Separate hard lumps, like nuts (hard to pass)
Type 2		Sausage-shaped but lumpy
Type 3		Like a sausage but with cracks on its surface
Type 4		Like a sausage or snake, smooth and soft
Type 5		Soft blobs with clear-cut edges (passed easily)
Type 6		Fluffy pieces with ragged edges, a mushy stool
Type 7		Watery, no solid pieces. **Entirely Liquid**

Reproduced with kind permission of Dr KW Heaton, formerly Reader in Medicine at the University of Bristol. ©2000, Norgine group of companies.

bowel movements per day to three per week is considered the normal range.

What's more important than frequency is the ease with which you move your bowels. If you need to push or strain, something is off. Many factors can affect regularity, such as diet, travel, medications, hormonal fluctuations, sleep patterns, exercise, and stress. The characteristics of your stool (the color, odor, shape, size) will tell you a good deal about how happy and healthy your digestive tract is.

So, let's look at the toilet bowl! The Bristol Stool Chart is a handy guide that may help you learn what you should be going for. Ideally, your stool should approximate Types 3, 4, and 5, "like a sausage or a snake, smooth and soft" to "soft blobs that pass easily." Type 4 is the ideal. If you regularly see these types of stools, your input is working for your system and being properly eliminated.

BACK PAIN AND CONSTIPATION

Analysis from the March–April 2008 Australian Longitudinal Study on Women's Health identified suggests a strong association between back pain and GI symptoms in women. The authors noted that potential reasons why the two issues go hand-in-hand include referred pain from the stomach into the back due to proximity, or viscerosomatic convergence, and increased spinal loading when straining to poop. I believe that men also suffer from this overlap in symptoms because my nutritional treatments result in great improvement in back pain for both genders.

POOP POINTERS

If you become constipated, you should eat fruits, vegetables, and other foods high in magnesium and fiber, such as beans and whole grains, and exercise to stimulate the bowels. A simple way to keep your GI tract on track is to drink a tall glass of cold water. This should help jump start your digestive and elimination systems. You should be drinking about 64 ounces or more of water per day to keep your digestive system happy.

WONDERFUL WATER

While different foods affect different stomachs differently, water is the one thing that all bodies need daily. Your stomach needs water to flush out the digestive system optimally. Good hydration is also essential for every cell and bodily function—from digestion to warding off sickness. Dehydration can cause a number of problems, such as fatigue and headaches, but also back pain. Why? Your vertebrae have discs between them that are composed of a jelly-like substance, which is 90 percent water. Lack of water causes the area around the spinal discs to become dry, and little fissures, or cracks, can form. If the fissures become severe, the inside of the discs can bulge and put pressure on your spinal nerves or spinal cord. Staying well-hydrated seems to help keep your back's cushioning intact. Many of my patients simply don't drink enough water. Coffee, iced tea, and beer do *not* constitute fluid and actually dehydrate you. You'll know you're well hydrated if your urine is clear to light yellow in color instead of dark yellow or brown like apple juice.

Retrieved from https://www.ncbi.nlm.nih.gov/pubmed/27412449

If you are having diarrhea, you should decrease your fiber intake and participate in a stress-reducing activity. If diarrhea is a recurring problem, consider food sensitivities or allergies as causes, and pay attention to how your bowels change after consuming certain foods. Of course, these are fixes for the occasional bout of an upset stomach. Back pain that is induced by digestive causes requires a greater change in your nutrition in order to affect your output and eliminate back pain. A happy digestive system is the key to a healthy, happy back!

THE LOWDOWN ON THOSE POOP "PROBLEM SOLVERS"

Just as there are always fads in diets, there are also fads in improving your output. Here are my thoughts on those so-called digestive solutions.

DITCH THE DETOXES

There has been much hoopla on cleanses, detox drinks, and juice fasts. I believe that the body already has a built-in detox system in the form of bowel movements. If your bowels are passing the test on the Bristol Stool Chart, there really is no need to detox because your body is already doing it. I would even go so far as to say that the cleanses and fasts may do more harm than good by being too rigorous and further upsetting the digestive system. Reducing inflammatory foods, eating healthful portions of food, which neither inundate your system nor starve it, and creating a meal and snack schedule to keep your digestive system and metabolism operating consistently, are the real keys to maintaining your natural detox function.

WHEN TO CAVE TO COLONICS

People frequently ask my opinion on colonics. I have personally never had one but have had patients who have had great relief from them. My recommendation is to use it as a last resort after you have tried to balance both the output and the input aspects of your digestive system. Colonics are great to clean you out, but ideally, you want to identify the cause of the imbalance.

THE PROBIOTIC PROMISE

Probiotics promise to help your digestive system get and stay on track, but probiotics work much in the same way as food—sometimes they are healthy for people, sometimes they are not! I have seen instances where they can be the cure of back pain—or the cause!

This is a story of a patient of mine named Rob, who is in his early forties and married with three kids. Rob leads quite an active lifestyle and travels extensively for work. One day, he came to me complaining of mid-back pain that just didn't seem to be going away. After treating the back pain structurally for a few weeks with manipulation, massage, heat, electrical stimulation, and stretches, the pain was still there. I therefore turned my attention to other factors: could it be his stress? He claimed that he felt pretty relaxed and that everything was really going great. I asked about his diet, and he said not much had changed since the onset of his pain, except that a few weeks ago, his wife saw a television show on the power of probiotics and started to give him one to take every morning. He then went on to say that the probiotic seemed to throw off his stomach a bit and gave him a bit of gas, but he kept taking it because it was supposed to be good for him. I told him what he said made sense, but if the probiotic was upsetting his stomach, it may not be helping him. I recommended that he stop taking the probiotic for two weeks and see how he felt. Not only did the gas go away, but the back pain did as well. The cause of Rob's back pain was actually his probiotic!

Conversely, I had a patient who was suffering from both lower back pain and an upset stomach but who ate a wide variety of non-inflammatory foods. Willow Jarosh, an expert nutritionist, recommended a probiotic to help balance my patient's stomach. Two weeks after taking the probiotic, my patient's stomach was calmed down, and her back pain was gone!

As you go through the Diagnostic Nutrition Test in Chapter 4 to assess your diet, keep in mind this rule of thumb: your body is unique and not just the same as anyone else's. What you eat and how your digestive system operates is also unique and may require a bit of a test run to help you identify what foods and supplements your body needs to operate optimally!

Principle 8.

Cut down on crap—but remember, you can have too much of a good thing!

Here is my list of "no-no's" that are consumed in high quantities and are known culprits of back pain!

Caffeine—Caffeine increases muscle contractions, which means that those back cramps or spasms could be caused by your daily cup of joe, especially if you find yourself consuming it in large doses.

Sugar and sweeteners—The average American consumes about 175 pounds of sugar each year—including about 600 cans of soda a year, which is equivalent to ten teaspoons of sugar or an equal amount of artificial sweetener per pop. Too much sugar not only increases the rate at which you excrete calcium, but it also can irritate the digestive system and cause back pain.

Foods that end in -ose—Start reading your food labels. You'll probably find that much of what you consume includes substances with names you probably can't pronounce. Food is primarily made up of the first four or five ingredient listed on the label, so pay attention to the order in which the ingredients are listed. Ingredients ending in -ose are sugars, and prepared foods and condiments are loaded with them.

Watch out for these other red-flag ingredients:

- **Hydrogenated or partially hydrogenated oils,** found in margarine and other common ingredients, were originally added by food companies to extend shelf life.
- **Trans-fats,** which are made when vegetable oils are exposed to hydrogen, solidify at room temperature. Unfortunately, they are detrimental to our health and are now being removed from many foods.
- **Interesterified fat,** which, on food labels, is called interesterified soybean or stated rich oil, has been shown to

lower HDL, or good cholesterol, increase blood glucose levels, and depress insulin.

- **Enriched wheat flour,** which is neither whole wheat nor oat bran flour, does not deliver the nutrients and fiber you need.
- **Other additives,** including those that end with *-ates* or *-ites*, as in nitrates and nitrites, are found in processed meats.
- **Food coloring** should be avoided, because it's an unnatural ingredient!
- **Tyramine,** a naturally occurring substance formed from the breakdown of protein as food ages, is found in alcoholic beverages, aged cheeses, and processed meats and has been associated with increased systolic blood pressure and migraines.

Another Patient's Story

ABOUT TEN YEARS AGO, while skiing in Utah with friends, I sat down on a bench and leaned over to buckle my ski boots when my back exploded. The pain was so bad I couldn't stand up and had to crawl on all fours. I was only forty years old and never had any issues with my back in my life! A friend of mine knew Dr. Sinett and told me to see him when I got back to New York. I scheduled an appointment for the following week, but I had to walk around with a cane until then.

When I met Dr. Sinett and told him what happened, one of the first things he asked me was, "Is there anything in your diet that is excessive?" At the time, I was addicted to Diet Coke. I would drink four 20-ounce bottles a day. Dr. Sinett said, "I will bet if you stop drinking Diet Coke, it will have a meaningful impact on your physical condition."

At the time, I had no knowledge that your diet could impact your back, but I would have tried anything, so I agreed to stop drinking it. Dr. Sinett then manipulated my stomach, putting his fingers in my abdominal area. It was very painful! He told me that this digestive issue would have shown up in some other way eventually; in my case, it showed up in back spasms and pain. I went for a follow-up visit and within three days of eliminating the soda, I was on my feet as if nothing had ever happened. Dr. Sinett explained that, although everyone is unique and everything should be taken in moderation, for me, the diet soda was poison. In fact, soda is one of the unhealthiest beverages.

What Dr. Sinett introduced to me was the idea that your physical health can be impacted by stress caused by any one of three factors: physical, emotional, or dietary. Since my back pain episode, I go to Dr. Sinett every three to four weeks on a proactive basis to get adjustments, manage stress, and stay attentive to my diet.

—*Gus Field*

What if too much crap isn't your problem? Well, there are also some healthy foods that cause digestive trouble when eaten repetitively:

- Salad
- Oatmeal
- Egg whites
- Tofu
- Smoothies

- Raw vegetables
- Frozen yogurt
- Beans
- Fresh-squeezed juices
- Protein bars

In these cases, too much roughage is the biggest culprit, causing your digestive tract to go into overdrive. Most things in moderation are okay, but you'll learn as you go through the diet and journaling process which foods, if any, are particularly inflammatory for your system and must be taken off your list of edibles.

Another Patient's Story

IN SEPTEMBER 2015, I was playing college hockey when I herniated a disc in my lower back and had a bulging disc. The injury was a result of wear and tear over time, and eventually my back gave out on me. A year and a half later, I still wasn't feeling quite like myself and received a recommendation from a family friend to see Dr. Sinett.

Dr. Sinett told me that my original injury had healed, but it seemed like other things were putting pressure on my lower back. He told me my digestive system was inflamed and asked about my diet. Once I started training seriously, I was taught to bring a protein shake to drink after a workout, and I packed in extra protein bars during and between my college classes. When I showed Dr. Sinett my weekly nutrition plan, he said I had been overloading my body. He told me to cut out the protein bars and shakes for a month and to simplify my diet. I followed his advice, eliminated the protein supplements, and stuck to eating real foods, such as meat with brown rice or quinoa, immediately after training sessions and throughout the day.

Sure enough, in a week, my stomach was less inflamed. I used to get bloated after drinking shakes, and suddenly, I felt less lethargic and healthier. I believed I was doing all the right things by following the approach I was taught in my health sessions for athletes. The protein bars and shakes were convenient, and I thought I was putting decent quality stuff in my body. For me, it wasn't working and was causing inflammation and pressure in my back, which was throwing my body out of balance. Once I started feeling healthier and better in terms of back pain, I ultimately had better performance in sports and training.

I shared the information I had learned from Dr. Sinett with people to whom I was close and had trained with. Some of them were surprised, as I originally was. I am fortunate enough to have been surrounded by good people who were educated in sports nutrition and found that protein supplements worked for both the majority of people and themselves. However, I did pass on the information to a friend who was suffering from similar issues, and after a visit to Dr. Sinett, he also found that the protein bars and shakes were causing digestive inflammation. I think that a lot of kids fall into the trap of believing that this type of nutrition works for everyone. However, because everyone is different, what works for the majority of people may not work for you. Often, we don't even notice that we are doing things that are detrimental to our health and body. I really thought my diet was helping me. For me, it took a serious injury to go see Dr. Sinett and learn more about my body.

—Kevin Lohan

Principle 9.

Anything that can cause digestive distress can affect the muscular system, resulting in back pain.

This concept goes back to the concept of interconnectedness in the body and the internal chain reaction that can happen when one part of the body becomes irritated. Patients with digestive-related disorders, such as irritable bowel syndrome, for example, frequently complain of low back pain. For those with no gastro-intestinal disorder, referred back pain can actually feel worse than the stomach ache and can truly become an example of what we often find, "The pain is not where the problem is."

GAS CAUSES BACK PAIN!

As we learned earlier, digestive dysfunction and problems with the ileocecal valve can create gas. Gas sounds a bit stinky but may not seem like a big deal. Yet it is! Back pain can sometimes be caused by excess gas in your gut. The trapped gas and bloating caused by digestive irritation creates swelling in the abdomen, putting pressure on the back and spine and resulting in lower or middle back pain. If these two symptoms seem to occur in tandem, your bloating may be giving rise to your lower back pain.

You may remember my patient Kevin Dailey, who described seeing large amounts of gas in the X-ray of his stomach. You'll see on the following page an example of an X-ray that exhibits a healthy stomach. There is a clear image of the spine and pelvic bones.

Now, compare this to the following X-rays of two people with substantial gas!

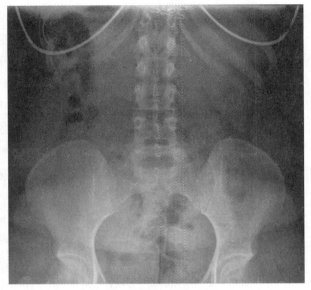

Healthy Stomach

Do you see all the circles, or gas bubbles, throughout the abdomen? The first X-ray (on the left) reveals moderate gas. In the x-ray on the right, there is so much gas that you can't get a good look at the patient's bones. But you certainly can see what is causing their discomfort!

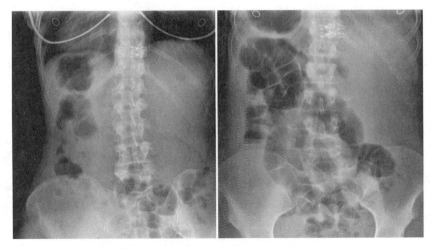

Moderate Gas   **Heavy Gas**

For gas to show up on an X-ray like this, there has to be about fourteen pounds of gas per square inch! For comparison's sake, a football (no Tom Brady jokes!) has about thirteen-and-a-half pounds of gas per square inch, while a basketball has seven-and-a-half pounds of gas per square inch. People are frequently walking around with gas pressure in their abdominal cavity that is equal to the pressure of an inflated football and don't even know it! They tend to think that it's normal because they are used to feeling that way. They may not even consider themselves "gassy" people, because the gas just gets trapped in the stomach and doesn't pass frequently. Interestingly enough, these people come to me complaining of back pain, not abdominal pain. Once you see this on an X-ray, however, you know that reducing the gas and inflammation in the gut is vital to ridding the patient of the back pain. Frequently, patients will only realize how uncomfortable they were digestively after a diet change eliminates the gas and bloating.

For me, the frustrating part is that radiologists will disregard these very clear X-ray findings, because they are trained to look only for fractures, tumors, diseases, and arthritis. That is why many doctors aren't diagnosing you correctly and are missing the diet connection completely!

CRAMPING YOUR STYLE

While not all muscle cramping is due to dietary factors, dehydration and magnesium deficiency seem to be the most influential in muscle cramping. Magnesium helps stabilize adenosine triphosphate (ATP), the energy source for muscle contraction, and also serves as an electrolyte in body fluids; therefore, when you suffer from magnesium deficiency, you are likely to have weakness, twitching, and cramps in your muscles. To help prevent muscle cramps, all of my back pain diets include foods rich in magnesium.

Principle 10.

Variety is vital. Mix it up by having at least three different types of breakfasts, lunches, and dinners, as well as snacks, in your rotation.

An apple a day may keep the doctor near. We all need variety in our diets. This gives our digestive system time to digest other foods. If you tend to eat a large amount of carbohydrates, the small intestine, responsible for digesting those foods, may become too taxed. Too much protein can overrun the stomach, which needs to produce acid to digest the proteins. Also, our bodies need a variety of nutrients that can't be gotten from just a few foods. For example, carrots contain different vitamins and nutrients than broccoli, and chicken is very different nutritionally than fish.

Another Patient's Story

A FEW YEARS AGO, I woke up with this pain that radiated from my right buttock down my leg and into my ankle. I had been seeing Dr. Sinett for several years, so I made an appointment with him and told him I thought I had developed sciatica. "Well, we'll see," Dr. Sinett said. He pressed on my stomach and asked, "What have you been eating?!"

I'm mainly a vegetarian, and I told him my meals consisted

of bowls of vegetable soup, flax bread, and lots of raw vegetables. He told me I was eating way too much fiber—it was bulking me up! And when he pressed on my stomach, he felt it! He spent some time manipulating my stomach and asked to see me two to three times a week for a while so that he could get my stomach moving. I didn't want to go to a nutritionist, and he told me all I had to do was simply "change it up."

Sure enough, I was able to do it on my own. Now, I still have salads but I don't overdo it. I limit my fruit to one or two pieces a day. I start my day with hard-boiled eggs and regular toast (I'm afraid to touch the fibrous flax bread!), or I might have an orange and almonds or gluten-free steel cut oats. Now, when I do go overboard with my vegetables, I'm conscious of it.

Changing my diet didn't mean getting rid of health food. I still drink water; never soda, and I don't eat a lot of processed foods. I make sure my diet is based on whole foods. It's been two years since I've "changed it up," and I've been free of pain.

—MaryAnn Simone

LISTEN TO YOUR BODY

Following these ten principles will help you learn to listen to your body. This sounds simple, but for many, it isn't. Just because your taste buds like something doesn't mean your stomach does. Your body knows what is good for it and what isn't; you just have to listen and obey. If you had Chinese food last night, and you didn't feel well this morning, ask yourself whether it was the three beers you had with dinner or the food itself. If you routinely get a stomach ache after consuming milk products, you might have lactose intolerance. If you really pay attention to your body's signals, you can avoid the things that upset your system and find relief in both your stomach and your back!

Part of listening to your body is realizing the effect your emotions and stress have on your digestive process. There is a completely different digestive process if you are eating a hot fudge sundae when you are celebrating than eating one when you are depressed. Food is meant to be eaten. Emotions are meant to be handled. Your emotional states and relationships with food need to be mutually supportive in order to regulate your digestive process and rid yourself of back pain. Not paying attention to this relationship is why many people end up with digestively induced back pain, weight gain from emotional eating, and other food-related issues. If your issues with food feel bigger than you are, a therapist might be helpful in starting this process. Sometimes, it's just about becoming more mindful of your body and its messages.

Another Patient's Story

THROUGHOUT COLLEGE AND GRAD school, I had a lot of stomach issues. I would eat something and swell up. I wasn't just getting bloated; I was constantly feeling sick and in pain. I knew my body was inflamed, and I knew I had a family history (my mom had also struggled with life-long stomach issues and ultimately was diagnosed with colitis), but I just didn't want to deal with it.

Eventually, my mom went gluten-free and found a lot of relief for her colitis. Because I thought I had issues similar to hers, I decided to go completely gluten-free and to try and avoid dairy myself. Over the next six months, I gained eleven pounds and didn't find any relief from my pain and puffiness. It only got worse. Finally, at age twenty-five, I went to a gastroenterologist. When my blood test for allergies came up negative, the doctor felt I should get a colonoscopy. My mother and I both felt I was too young and was sure diet and nutrition was my problem. But this doctor made me paranoid, so I did both a colonoscopy and an endoscopy. When she called with the results, she said the endoscopy showed acid reflux, and the colonoscopy showed that my colon was "damaged." She suggested ulcerative colitis was likely or that there was possible scarring from too much pain medication (Advil, ibuprofen) or from a previous virus or infection. I sobbed, thinking there was something really wrong with me.

I decided to get a second opinion. I brought the results of my colonoscopy to a different doctor, who said that not only was my colon not damaged, but it was totally normal. This doctor felt I had IBS, which was more in line with what I had been feeling when I first sought help.

But now, I was confused and upset. I didn't know what to do.

Meanwhile, my parents had been seeing Dr. Sinett and raved about him. I was hesitant, because I thought chiropractors were just a quick fix. But my parents were insistent that Dr. Sinett could help me with everything—even my stress and anxiety, which seemed to be exacerbating my stomach distress. My dad made an appointment for me. I told Dr. Sinett about my gluten-free diet and subsequent weight gain and explained how uncomfortable, swollen, and puffy I felt. I also had developed lower back pain in the recent months, along with a worsening of the plantar fasciitis in my feet.

Dr. Sinett did a physical check and saw that I had an

imbalance in my feet, but he also did X-rays and saw a lot of gas. He felt we had to start with my diet, because my stomach was my biggest complaint. I was eating a lot of salads with my gluten-free diet (probably five days out of the week!), and he wanted me to reduce my salad intake and cut out coffee (I typically had one to two cups a day). Giving up coffee was hard! I was cranky and irritable for about two weeks; I couldn't sleep, and I had headaches. But Dr. Sinett was sure that the coffee was irritating my whole system and that anything I ate would give me pain until my system was soothed. So, I powered through, and very quickly, I noticed a difference. Even my face was back to normal—not puffy at all! I lost the eleven pounds I had gained instantly. My mood changed. Amazingly, I wasn't doing anything else differently; I had just reduced the inflammation in my body.

Once my system was finally cleared, I could eat certain foods and tell right away what was hurting me. For example, having cutting out salads, I drank a carrot-ginger-kale juice and swelled up immediately. If I have a big salad now, it gives me terrible cramps and sends me running to the bathroom. Before meeting Dr. Sinett, I never would have thought that the gluten-free diet was bad for me. I thought I was eating healthy! I learned I benefit from a turkey sandwich much more than a kale salad. Kale is actually the worst food for my body. And that was my biggest lesson from Dr. Sinett: everybody is different, and every person has different needs. The roughage and the acid from coffee are the things that are bad for me.

I still eat vegetables, but I cook them. I incorporate small salads, take a multivitamin, and eat a lot of salmon, chicken, rice, and whole grains. When I eat, I listen to my body, and if I feel pain, it's a reminder of what I should avoid. Stress can really affect my stomach as well, and I meet with a stress manager at Dr. Sinett's office often. Sometimes, I'll have a glass of wine and feel great; sometimes, I'll have a glass and feel sick. Dr. Sinett taught me that drinking when you are happy can have a very different effect on your body than drinking when you are stressed. The food irritant coupled with the stress can seriously affect your health. These lessons—Don't Follow the Trends, and Listen to Your Body—have guided my life and brought me back to health.

—*Sarah LaFontaine*

A MORSEL ON INTUITIVE EATING

As we begin this journey to back health via nutrition, it's important to pay attention to a new fad in dieting, which is, interestingly, the anti-diet known as Intuitive Eating. Intuitive eating basically means tuning into your body's hunger signals to help control weight. Gaining awareness of your own actual hunger helps you overcome mindless eating, eating from boredom, and eating from emotional stress, among other things. You are therefore only eating when your body is actually in need of nourishment, and you thereby reduce all the excess munching that leads to weight gain. Overeating is one factor that leads to stomach inflammation, as the digestive system gets inundated with more than it can efficiently process. Here are a few tips to keep you from overeating:

- Eat something within one hour of getting up each morning to jumpstart your metabolism and keep you from getting too hungry by mid-morning.

- Have a healthful snack between meals each day to keep your stomach from going on empty, and reduce what you eat in one sitting during meals.
- Your hunger level should determine your portions. Going too long between eating and feeling starved or overeating and feeling stuffed not only affects your digestive system and moods, but it also affects the back. The "hangries" can take on a whole new meaning if your diet causes your back pain. On a hunger scale with one being famished and ten being stuffed, you want to eat when you are at a level three and stop when you are at a level six. Willow, the nutritionist, likes to use "the treadmill test": at any point, you should be able to go on a treadmill and exercise and not be impeded by being either too full or too famished. This will allow you to feel engaged and energized all day without having large blood sugar swings that will lead to crashes.
- Eat slowly to allow yourself to be aware of feeling full.
- If overeating is your problem, try to leave a little bit on your plate at each meal. It's a good way to slowly start reducing your intake.
- Keep a food journal. Sometimes you don't realize how much all that grazing adds up until you see it on paper.

It's always amazing when my patients comment that they didn't realize they were feeling stomach discomfort until *after* they started feeling better. Most people are eating not only without paying enough attention to hunger but also without paying enough attention to their body's other signals, like pain, bloating, gas, discomfort, and the quality of their bowel movements. Intuitive eating is essential in many ways as you go through the nutrition plans that follow. I've found that overeating can contribute to digestive distress, and listening to your own hunger can be the first step in modifying your eating habits in a healthier direction. It's also necessary to become supremely conscious of your body's signals after eating, and use those to help guide your choices the next time it's time to eat. The Symptom Journal included at the end of the book can help you track your body's signals both before and after meals until intuitive eating becomes more natural to you.

A lot of people don't realize that the body generally likes to have structure around mealtimes, and my meal plans create a meal and snack routine that both meets your nutritional needs and follows the ideal rhythm of the metabolism. I find starting with a guided nutrition plan gives you the visual for what a day should look like and offers a starting point for how much to eat at a time. Of course, there's always an adjustment based on size, physical activity, and more, and this is where your own intuitive eating should really kick in. The most important thing for you to do is to be aware not only of how much and when you are eating, but also in this case, to take better inventory of your body's other digestive signals in addition to hunger.

3.

HOW MUCH OF YOUR PAIN IS DIGESTIVE?

Now you are armed with your ten principles and our new, three-pronged motto: **we are what we eat, we are what we digest,** and **we are what we can properly excrete.** What you eat—whether it's too much coffee, too many sweets, or a host of other edibles that have a unique impact on you—can agitate your digestive system and chemically induce back pain.

In order to determine if what you are eating is a significant cause of your back pain, the following questions will help you assess the digestive and hormonal factors that may be causing inflammation in one or more parts of your body.

THE DIGESTIVE INFLAMMATION TEST

When a patient has dietary issues, we look for either changes in the chemical system or repetitive patterns that can result in back pain. Hormonal changes also fall into the digestive/chemical category and can profoundly influence back health.

Answer **YES** *or* **NO** *to each question, giving* **one point** *for* **yes** *and* **zero points** *for* **no**.

_____ Have you been constipated recently?

_____ Have you had diarrhea recently?

_____ Has your stomach been bothering you?

_____ Have you had an increase in gas?

_____ Have you eaten any types of food that you don't normally consume?

_____ Have you eaten spicy foods recently?

_____ Have you recently had a stomach virus?

_____ Have you been on any new medication(s)?

_____ Have you changed your diet?

_____ Have you changed your vitamin regimen?

_____ Have you increased your fiber intake?

_____ Do you tend to have the same meals more than three times in a week?

_____ Do you eat five large raw salads or more in a week?

_____ Have you recently started to drink five or more fruit smoothies in a week?

_____ Are you taking more than three different vitamins in a day?

_____ Have you recently become a vegetarian?

_____ Do you eat five or more cups of fruits and vegetables in a day?

_____ Have you recently started to drink something different?

_____ Have you drunk more than four alcoholic beverages in one sitting in the past week?

_____ Do you depend on coffee or soda to stay awake during the day?

_____ Do you have coffee at least once a day?

_____ Are you having more than three protein bars in a week?

_____ Do you use protein bars as meal replacements?

_____ Do you eat more than one small dessert or treat during the day?

_____ Do you use an artificial sweetener?

_____ Do you have regular bowel movements?

_____ Have you been diagnosed with IBS (Irritable Bowel Syndrome)?

_____ Do you turn to food when you're stressed or upset?

_____ Do you skip meals?

_____ Do you ever eat when you're not hungry or continue eating after you are full?

_____ Do you eat at your desk?

_____ Did you just begin your menstrual period, or have you recently started menopause?

_____ Has your hormonal system undergone any recent changes (menopause, change in birth control, missed menstrual period, pregnancy, etc.)?

Add up the number of times you answered "yes."

SCORING YOUR STOMACH

4 POINTS OR LESS

If you answered "yes" fewer than four times, you are at low risk for a digestive cause of back pain. Your cause is likely structural and/or emotional. I suggest looking at my book *3 Weeks to a Better Back* to help you best focus your attention on the more likely causes of your back pain and find at-home treatment options. A local chiropractor also may be helpful in treating your structural pain, and a therapist may offer stress-coping mechanisms to help improve your daily life.

5 TO 10 POINTS

If you answered "yes" between five and ten times, you are at moderate risk for digestively induced back pain, which means digestive issues are probably contributing to your back pain. You will very likely find some relief by using my guide to digestive solutions found in Chapter 4 in order to identify some of your trigger foods and by following one of the nutrition plans to reduce your internal inflammation.

MORE THAN 10 POINTS

If you answered "yes" more than ten times, your back pain most definitely has a digestive root. "Digestive Solutions," as outlined in Chapter 4, will help you begin your digestive evaluation and find the right nutrition plan to help reduce your stomach and back pain.

HOW DEEP DOES DIGESTION GO?

To further help you understand the diet/pain connection, here are two patients' stories to illustrate what your pain might be like if you scored either in the five-to-ten-points bracket or in the more-than-ten-points bracket on the Digestive Inflammation Test. Richard is a patient of mine who found that both diet and structural causes were causing his back pain. Reducing sugar and caffeine, in addition to utilizing structural treatments, helped rid him of his pain. One treatment would not have been sufficient in resolving both causes.

One Patient's Story

I WAS LIVING AND working in Japan in early 2014 when I started getting various pains in my leg. I thought it was my hamstring and went to physical therapy as well as saw a few chiropractors in Tokyo. It made some impact, but not enough, and eventually the pain spread. I tried acupuncture without any success and had a series of cortisone injections in my back. For the next year, I muddled through with a lot of pain; I couldn't play squash or do any significant physical activity. In July 2015, I repatriated to the United States.

In October of that year, I experienced the most pain I'd ever been in. I had just suffered a back spasm that left me barely able to move. I was actually unable to put on my socks. At that time, I was referred to Dr. Sinett. Dr. Sinett had me use his Backbridge and did his adjustments and electric stimulation therapy, but he felt there might be a missing piece. He asked me about my stress, and we ultimately determined stress wasn't causing my back pain. He turned toward diet, and straightaway asked about my intake of caffeine and sugar. I told him I had one tall coffee each morning and one cup a couple of afternoons a week, and he asked me to cut out all caffeine. I spent some time after that with his nutritionist doing weekly food charts, writing down my diet day by day, and I began an elimination diet to see if there was something specific I was allergic to. The conclusion was that although I wasn't allergic to something specific, eating healthier and more cleanly would help me eliminate some of the inflammation I had in my gut.

In addition to cutting out the caffeine, Dr. Sinett felt that I should reduce the sugar in my diet. At first, I resisted, because I didn't want to take alcohol completely out of my diet, and that has sugar. However, by the start of 2015, I agreed to try it for thirty days and cut out pasta, rice, desserts, and alcohol. Thirty days turned into one hundred days. That did the most benefit in resetting my stomach, which had taken years of abuse, and in stabilizing my back. Now I eat sugar and drink alcohol in moderation, but I've managed to avoid the caffeine.

Now, I am aware of the impact of my diet on my body. When I indulge a little bit, it's fine. When I indulge a lot, I have to be more careful.

In all my treatments prior to meeting Dr. Sinett, no one else had considered diet as a factor in my back pain. However, if I'd only done the diet, I wouldn't have recovered, and I wouldn't have recovered without changing my diet. Eating differently was the missing element of my treatment, and in conjunction with the structural solutions, this combination has gotten me back to golfing and working out three to four times a week.

—Richard S.

Another Patient's Story

HERE'S WHAT HAPPENED TO another patient who definitely scored more than ten points on the Digestive Inflammation Test:

One Saturday afternoon, I received a call from a Grammy-winning recording artist who was suffering from severe upper back and neck pain. Her pain was so bad that she couldn't turn her neck and was concerned that she wasn't going to be able to make it through her performance on *Saturday Night Live* nor a concert that was scheduled for the following day.

I examined her and noticed her whole muscular system was tight, almost to the point of rigidity, as if she were suffering from a full-body spasm. I also could tell she was experiencing severe gas pains, and she revealed to me that her on-the-road diet was full of fast and processed foods. I immediately knew the root of her problem.

The good news was we had a diagnosis—back pain stemming from an inflamed digestive system—and a solution—a healthy nutrition plan. The bad news was I couldn't cure her immediately. When a physical reaction is that severe, it reflects a toxic buildup within the body, a situation that requires both a reorientation of the diet and time for the body to self-cleanse and readjust. I've seen many cases like this, especially when patients say they don't have much time to prepare meals. My "healthy eaters" often suffer from gassiness, bloating, stomach pain, and bouts of both diarrhea and constipation. In the next chapter, "Proper Foods for Your Digestive System," you will learn first to identify your triggers and then how to best treat your digestive system.

PART II

PROPER FOODS AND PRACTICAL MEAL PLANS

4.

PROPER FOODS FOR YOUR DIGESTIVE SYSTEM

If anti-inflammatory medications have been prescribed and are proven to reduce back pain, why then can't an anti-inflammatory diet do the same thing? **The fact is, it can.**

Some foods are known to be inflammatory and other foods are anti-inflammatory. For example, caffeine, alcohol, and sugar are part of many people's daily diet and these substances have been shown to increase cortisol levels. Cortisol is a chemical produced by the body in response to stress and to low blood-glucose concentration. When too much cortisol is present in your system, connective tissue throughout the body can become inflamed, causing pain.

Eating right counteracts the inflammatory process in the body. To find the underlying chemical cause of pain, the first step is to determine whether there have been changes in your eating pattern that would alter the chemical system, or whether you have developed repetitive eating patterns that have become toxic and, over time, have broken down the body's natural resistance. This may include eating too much of a "good thing," such as raw fruits and vegetables and other roughage. As we figure out the right nutrition solution for you, you'll want to think about your pain pattern and see if you can trace your pain to poor dietary choices that also may have resulted in reflux, gas pains, diarrhea, or constipation. Proper foods for your system will be the best medicine you can get!

TAKING THE "DIAGNOSTIC NUTRITION TEST"

If you scored five or more points on the Digestive Inflammation Test in the previous chapter, the next step is to find the underlying nutritional cause of pain. You will be able to do this by taking the Diagnostic Nutrition Test below. Based on your score and answers, you will know which back pain relief diet to try. Each diet is designed for a specific reason, but the purpose of all the diets is cutting down the inflammation in your digestive system in order to eliminate your back pain.

For some, the solution may be quite easy and clear. For others, we may have to dig deep into your diet. Suffice it to say, the assessment test should put you on the right path.

THE DIAGNOSTIC NUTRITION TEST

Take this quiz to find out what plan you should follow first. From the multiple choices below each question, select one to answer as honestly as you can. If you are having trouble deciding between two answers, skip the question and come back to it once you've answered the other questions.

FOOD/BEVERAGE HABITS

1. *How often do you drink caffeinated beverages (coffee, soda, etc.)?*
   a. At least two times per day—I need it to start my day and get through the afternoon.
   b. Once per day in the morning—it helps keep me regular in addition to giving me energy.
   c. Occasionally to never—I can take or leave them.

2. *How often do you drink alcohol?*
   a. More than one to two drinks daily or binge drinking (which is more than three drinks per day) at least once a week.
   b. One drink daily to a few times a week.
   c. Occasionally (once per week) to never.

3. *I tend to crave sweet foods on a regular basis.*
   a. Always.
   b. Sometimes.
   c. I usually stay away from added sugar.

4. *Do you eat processed foods (white flour crackers/ bread, energy bars, pre-made meals, etc.)?*
   a. More than once a day.
   b. About once daily.
   c. Fewer than three times each week to never.

5. *Do dairy foods cause you any discomfort?*
   a. None; I can eat all dairy foods.
   b. They make me bloated/give me stomach cramps/cause diarrhea.
   c. None, but I don't eat a lot of dairy.

6. *Do gluten-containing foods cause you any discomfort?**
   a. None; I eat gluten regularly.
   b. I think they do, but I had a celiac test, and it was negative.
   c. None, but I don't eat a lot of gluten.

7. *How often do you eat RAW vegetables?*
   a. I eat them sometimes but haven't noticed whether they give me digestive upset.
   b. I prefer cooked veggies. Raw veggies don't sit well with me.
   c. I eat mostly raw veggies, and they don't give me any problems with digestion.

* If you've tested positive for celiac disease, a strict gluten-free diet is necessary. If you have been experiencing gastrointestinal symptoms and haven't yet had a test for celiac disease, we recommend speaking to your doctor about ruling this disease out.

8. *Do you eat cereals, energy bars, protein powder, or other foods with added fiber?*
    a. Sometimes.
    b. Never.
    c. Many of the packaged foods I eat have added fiber.

9. How much fruit do you eat daily?
    a. It varies from day to day, and I don't really keep track.
    b. One to two pieces.
    c. Three or more, sometimes in the form of fruit juice.

YOUR BODY

10. *Do you ever have irritated skin and/or rashes?*
    a. Never.
    b. I struggle with these on a regular basis.
    c. Rarely.

11. *How often do you experience diarrhea/constipation and/or bloating?*
    a. Very rarely for all three.
    b. On a weekly basis (or more often), and I'm least bloated right after a bowel movement.
    c. I rarely experience constipation, but I do get bloated several times a month.

12. *How do you feel right after you eat?*
    a. Fine.
    b. Bloated and gassy.
    c. Full, but the feeling goes away quickly.

13. *How often do you have a bowel movement?*

    a. Every one to two days.

    b. Varies widely.

    c. Daily.

14. *In terms of my weight,*

    a. I'm actively trying to lose weight.

    b. I want to be a healthy weight but am most concerned with fixing my digestive discomfort.

    c. I'm happy with my weight.

YOUR LIFESTYLE

15. *How would you describe your stress level?*

    a. Pretty normal—I don't really think about it much.

    b. High—I feel stressed almost all the time.

    c. Moderate—I feel stressed regularly (at least once a day).

*Now, add up the number of **A's** (___), the number of **B's** (___), and the number of **C's** (___) you gave yourself.*

WHICH MEAL PLAN SHOULD I FOLLOW?

In the next chapter, you will choose from among three, successful back pain relief diets. The guidelines below will help you know which diet to follow.

MY ANSWERS WERE MOSTLY A'S

If you answered mostly A's, it seems you may be eating too many processed foods for your body and may have some sensitivity to dairy and gluten. You will start with your choice of the **No-More-Back-Pain Diet** *or* the **Paleo Plus Meal Plan** (which is an alternative to the same diet). Both diets are whole-foods-based and are balanced with protein, carbs, and healthy fats.

I like to give patients a choice of diets, because a new diet or a change in diet can be a very hard thing for people to adjust to. Here, whereas the No-More-Back-Pain Diet is a looser guide to eating, and includes suggested meals, the Paleo Plan is a more regimented version of this same diet and includes detailed recipes. If you find that something more regimented is more helpful in the beginning to get you on track, start with the Paleo. If that scares you away, and you need a bit more flexibility to prevent you from ditching it altogether, do the No-More-Back-Pain Diet. Take a look at both plans, and choose your path. And if you struggle with one, or conversely find relief, you can continue by experimenting with foods or recipes from both diets!

MY ANSWERS WERE MOSTLY B'S

If you answered mostly B's, you will follow the **FODMAPS Diet**. This is an elimination diet to help with the symptoms of Irritable

Bowel Syndrome (IBS) and is low in fermentable oligo-, di-, and monosaccharides and polyols (FODMAPs). That means you will be limiting foods that contain:

- Lactose—found in milk, ice cream, yogurt, and cheese
- Fructose—found in fruits such as apples, pears, peaches, mangos, and berries
- Fructans—found in wheat, onions, garlic, asparagus, cauliflower, and mushrooms
- Galactans—found in beans and lentils
- Sugar alcohols (polyols)— found in honey, agave, high-fructose corn syrup, sorbitol, mannitol, Splenda, and other sweeteners.

These compounds in food can be poorly absorbed, leading to increased water and gas in the GI tract, and thus distention, bloating, and discomfort.

MY ANSWERS WERE MOSTLY C'S

If you answered mostly C's, you will follow **Digestive Rest**. This diet is best for those who have been eating too much of a good thing. It will help your body recover from inflammation caused by too much roughage and give your intestines a much-needed break from all things raw. The only thing it will allow is a little bit of fruit, which, in small doses, is a good digestive primer. However, you will be able to continue eating "health food." The diet will just help you make the shift to foods such as cooked vegetables, which are gentler on your system.

5.

HOW TO FOLLOW THE MEAL PLANS

Your answers on the Diagnostic Nutrition Test in Chapter 4 will help you select one of the three diets and meal plans that you will find in this chapter. You also can review all of the diets before beginning.

1. **Choose your plan.** Pick the best plan for you based on the test results. *Because each of the three diets in this book addresses a different aspect of potential digestive unrest, you may try one and find instant relief, or you may find that it takes two or even all three of the diets to discover what helps get your digestive system back into balance.*

   The FODMAPS plan eliminates specific carbohydrate triggers, meaning there will be certain grains, fruit, and veggies that are on the "do not eat" list, because they contain carbohydrates that your body cannot digest. The Paleo Plus and the No-More-Back-Pain diet plans help you get back into a healthy eating rhythm if you've turned to processed foods, skimp on produce, and use caffeine as your daily energy source. Finally, the Digestive Rest plans support soothing your digestive system by using only cooked vegetables, not going overboard with fruit, and making sure that high fiber foods are always balanced with other foods at meals so that your digestive system doesn't get an overload of fiber. If your score puts you evenly between two diet plans, which may happen, choose either one. If your symptoms are greatly reduced, but not gone, after trying the first diet, transition to the second one.

2. **Prep ahead.** With the exception of the first two-week plan, each plan is a full week of meals, snacks, and treats that cater to helping alleviate your specific symptoms. Each plan is designed to be followed in the order given (Day 1, Day 2, etc.) to make grocery shopping and prep work more efficient. We've incorporated into each plan reusing ingredients and utilizing leftovers so you're not cooking all day or wasting any food. If, however, you do need to eat the meals out of order, or repeat a day or two, that is completely fine. We recommend starting on a weekend when you have time to shop for groceries and clear out all the food you've been eating that seems to be triggering the problems!

3. **Keep a symptom journal.** You'll use this to describe your symptoms throughout the day on a scale from zero (nonexistent) to ten (severe). Keep your symptom journal wherever it is most convenient for you: on your phone notes, in an email, on your digital calendar, or on a calendar printout.

SUPER-FOODS: THE NUTRITIONIST'S CHOICE!

Throughout the following meal plans, you will see the repetition of certain foods included in the recipes. These foods tend to be easy on the stomach (although there is always the exception, so be sure to use that symptom journal). Repeated foods are highly nutritious and can be good substitute for things that you might be removing from your diet!

Almond milk. For people who can't fully digest dairy milk, almond milk steps in to lend a rich, creamy, smooth consistency to foods and drinks such as cereal, smoothies, and lattes. Most brands of almond milk are fortified with the same amount of calcium and vitamin D that you'll find in cow's milk, but all lack the protein of cow's milk. Therefore, be sure to include protein-rich foods in the meals where you use almond milk!

Dark chocolate. Treats are an important part of maintaining a balanced, healthy, enjoyable way of eating. Dark chocolate is packed with antioxidants, tastes delicious, and is really versatile in making creative desserts.

Eggs. Eggs are a simple, delicious way to add protein to a meal. Traditionally, they're used at breakfast, but a frittata or an omelet can be a fast, nutritious lunch or dinner, too. Also, using hard-boiled eggs is a simple way to add protein to snacks.

Avocado. This creamy fruit is a fantastic substitute for cheese when you're cutting out dairy to see if you're sensitive to it. Because of the creamy texture, it can be blended into salad dressings, used in smoothies, and spread onto sandwiches.

Nuts/seeds. We use an assortment of nuts and seeds in this plan, because they're loaded with a variety of nutrients, from zinc to omega-3 fatty acids. Getting a variety of nuts and seeds is best, since they each deliver a slightly different assortment of nutrients. In addition, eating nuts and seeds is a great way to add crunchy texture to dishes!

Sweet potatoes. Sweet potatoes are packed with vitamin A, which is a powerful antioxidant. They are also a really versatile high-fiber carbohydrate to add to breakfast, lunch, or dinner. Plus, you can cook them ahead of time, and they keep well in the fridge for easy additions to meals during busy weeks.

The No-More-Back-Pain Diet

■

If you scored mostly A's on the Diagnostic Nutrition Test, then the No-More-Back-Pain Diet is your first of two diet options. It has been designed to target and eliminate certain toxins from your system. It will make a dramatic difference in the way your body functions and how you feel, both in your back and throughout the rest of your body. The menu, or meal plan, is easy to put together and doesn't even require extensive recipes; it is more of a guide to what to eat on the plan. You should start with the full two-week plan to cleanse your system, and try to stick to the plan as best you can as you move forward. If you find you've eaten poorly at a party or during a vacation, following three to four days of the diet can help you reset your system after a short period of "going off the rails."

APPROVED FOODS

The foods in this plan may seem a little bland or plain, but this diet will give your stomach the break it needs!

- Whole grains, including whole grain breads, pastas, cereals, tortillas, and baked goods (look for the words whole grain on the food label followed by the name of the grain, such as wheat, corn, rice, oats, barley, quinoa, sorghum, and rye)

- Nuts and seeds, including nut and seed oils, nut and seed butters, unsweetened coconut, vegetable oils, olive oil, and flaxseed oil
- Protein, including chicken; fish (especially mackerel, lake trout, herring, sardines, albacore tuna, and salmon); lean cuts of meat (turkey, pork, beef); eggs
- Aged cheese
- Unsweetened non-dairy milk (almond, cashew, hemp, etc.), except soy
- Fermented dairy (yogurt and kefir)
- Vegetables, all, including starchy vegetables such as sweet potatoes, potatoes, corn, butternut squash, and peas
- Fruit
- Decaffeinated coffee and tea (unsweetened)
- Seltzer water, plain and flavored (however, the only ingredients should be water and natural flavor)
- Water

NON-APPROVED FOODS

Elimination of these foods will help rid your body of certain toxins and help your digestive system rest:

- Enriched white flour and products made from it, commonly found in breads, pasta, biscuits, waffles, crackers, muffins, cereal, pancakes, croutons, rolls, pretzels, graham crackers, cookies, baked goods, and tortillas

- Hydrogenated oils (look for the words *trans-fat, partially hydrogenated oil,* and *hydrogenated oil* on the food label)*
- Processed cheese or cheese products (only aged cheeses or fermented dairy such as kefir and yogurt is allowed)
- Dairy milk
- All sweetened beverages, artificially-flavored and/or sweetened fruit drinks)*
- All fruit juice
- Soft drinks, including diet sodas*
- Wine, beer, spirits, and cordials
- Caffeinated coffee and tea

* Added sweeteners, including sugar, molasses, honey, agave nectar, and artificial sweeteners, and products made with them

THE NO-MORE-BACK-PAIN MEAL PLAN

DAY 1

Breakfast

- ► 1 cup whole grain, no-sugar-added cereal, like shredded wheat, with ½ cup unsweetened almond milk
- ► ½ cup fruit
- ► ¾ cup plain yogurt with cinnamon
- ► 1 cup decaffeinated herbal tea

Lunch

- ► 1 grilled cheese sandwich: 1 ounce aged cheddar cheese on 2 slices whole grain bread toasted in 1 tsp olive oil
- ► 1 mixed salad: 1 cup mixed greens, ⅓ cup sliced cucumber, and ⅓ cup diced tomato; 2 tsp olive oil and 2 tsp vinegar for dressing

Dinner

- ► 2 cups steamed veggies with 1 tsp butter or olive oil
- ► 4 ounces broiled filet mignon (preferably grass-fed)
- ► 1 baked potato topped with 2 tbsp plain yogurt and chives

DAY 2

Breakfast

- ► 2 scrambled eggs
- ► 2 pieces whole grain toast with 2 tsp butter

- ▶ 1 cup fresh fruit
- ▶ 1 cup decaf herbal tea

Lunch

- ▶ 1 grilled chicken sandwich: 1, 4-ounce grilled chicken breast, 1 whole grain hamburger roll, 2 tsp mayonnaise (or hummus), and lettuce and tomato

Dinner

- ▶ 1 cup diced roasted chicken (breast or thigh)
- ▶ 1 medium Russet or gold potato, roasted with 2 tsp olive oil
- ▶ 1 cup steamed green beans with lemon juice

DAY 3

Breakfast

- ▶ 1 whole grain frozen waffle topped 2 tbsp plain yogurt
- ▶ ½ of a banana, sliced, for topping the waffle
- ▶ 1 cup decaf herbal tea

Lunch

- ▶ 1 baked potato topped with ½ cup marinara, no sugar added, and ½ cup cooked ground turkey breast
- ▶ 1 cup veggie, such as broccoli, steamed or sautéed with 1 tbsp olive oil

Dinner

- ► Chicken soup with veggies and brown rice: 2 cups of chicken broth mixed with 4 ounces diced roasted chicken, 1 cup cooked rice, ½ cup diced carrots, and 1 cup baby spinach

DAY 4

Breakfast

- ► 1 whole wheat bagel spread with 2 tbsp nut butter
- ► 1 cup fresh fruit
- ► 1 cup decaf herbal tea

Lunch

- ► 1 turkey sandwich: 4 ounces nitrate-free turkey, 2 slices whole wheat bread with 2 tsp mayonnaise and mustard if desired

Dinner

- ► 1 bowl of whole grain or brown rice pasta tossed with ½ cup tuna or 3 ounces salmon, 2 tsp olive oil, and 1 cup cooked mixed vegetables (any kind)

DAY 5

Breakfast

- ▶ 1 egg plus 2 egg whites, scrambled in 1 tsp of olive oil
- ▶ 1 slice whole grain toast with 1 tsp butter
- ▶ ½ grapefruit

Lunch

- ▶ 1 grilled chicken salad: 2 cups mixed greens and raw veggies of choice, topped with 4 ounces grilled chicken or tuna; 2 tbsp oil and vinegar for dressing

Dinner

- ▶ 1½ cups whole grain pasta tossed with 1 tbsp olive oil, 1 tbsp aged Parmesan cheese, and crushed fresh garlic to taste
- ▶ 1 cup grilled or steamed mixed vegetables with ⅓ cup white beans

DAY 6

Breakfast

- ▶ 1 cup plain yogurt
- ▶ 1 cup cantaloupe
- ▶ 1 slice whole grain toast with 1 tsp nut butter

Lunch

- 1 slice whole grain bread topped with nitrate-free sliced turkey breast, lettuce, tomato, and 2 tsp mayonnaise
- 1 cup low-fat cottage cheese

Dinner

- 3 to 4 ounces sirloin steak, grilled or broiled
- 1 baked sweet potato topped with 1 tsp butter and cinnamon to taste
- 1 cup steamed broccoli or mixed veggies

DAY 7

Breakfast

- 1 cup plain cooked oats (old-fashioned rolled) with ½ cup diced apple and 1 tbsp crushed walnuts, sprinkled with cinnamon

Lunch

- Mixed greens with assorted veggies, topped with lean turkey, ham and aged cheddar cheese, and drizzled with 2 tbsp oil and vinegar dressing
- 1 very small whole grain roll or 1 slice whole grain bread

Dinner

- 1 broiled chicken breast, seasoned with lemon, garlic, onions, and parsley
- Mixed vegetables (roasted with 1 tbsp olive oil)
- ½ cup cooked brown rice or quinoa

DAY 8

Breakfast

- ▶ 1 whole grain English muffin topped with 1 poached egg, 1 slice Canadian bacon or smoked salmon, and sliced tomato
- ▶ 1 apple, sliced and sprinkled with cinnamon

Lunch

- ▶ 1 roasted vegetable sandwich: ½ cup roasted mixed veggies and 1 slice aged cheddar cheese, served on 2 slices of whole grain bread spread with 2 tbsp hummus

Dinner

- ▶ 6 ounces lean ground turkey or beef (at least 94 percent lean) mixed with unsweetened tomato sauce and veggies (onions, peppers, and mushrooms)
- ▶ 1½ cups of cooked whole wheat or brown rice pasta

DAY 9

Breakfast

- ▶ Oatmeal with 2 tbsp chopped walnuts and a sliced pear, sprinkled with cinnamon
- ▶ ½ cup unsweetened almond milk

Lunch

- 1 chef's salad: mixed greens, roasted turkey, roasted ham, aged cheddar cheese, and mixed raw vegetables, dressed with 2 tbsp oil and vinegar dressing
- 1 whole wheat English muffin with 2 tbsp hummus

Dinner

- 4 ounces roasted pork tenderloin sprinkled with sea salt and chili powder
- 1 medium baked sweet potato topped with cinnamon and a dollop of plain yogurt
- 1 cup broccoli sautéed in garlic and 1 tsp olive oil

DAY 10

Breakfast

- 1 whole grain bagel or 1 slice of whole grain bread with 1 tbsp almond butter
- 6 ounces plain yogurt with ½ cup mixed frozen organic berries, sprinkled with cinnamon

Lunch

- ¾ cup cooked lentils mixed with ¾ cup quinoa, 1 cup baby spinach, and 2 tbsp crushed peanuts topped with ½ cup roasted and seasoned grilled tofu

Dinner

- ► 1, 4-ounce poached chicken breast
- ► 1 cup cooked brown rice
- ► 1½ cups purple cabbage sautéed in 2 tsp olive oil
- ► 1 cup diced potato roasted in 2 tsp olive oil

DAY 11

Breakfast

- ► 1 cup unsweetened whole grain flake cereal mixed with ½ cup puffed wheat cereal
- ► ½ cup low-fat or unsweetened almond milk
- ► ½ cup sliced strawberries
- ► 2 tbsp sliced or slivered unsalted almonds

Lunch

- ► 1 avocado and black bean roll-up: 1 whole grain tortilla spread with thin layer of yogurt, ¼ of an avocado, 1 cup black beans, and 2 tbsp salsa
- ► 1 cup cucumber slices drizzled with 1 tsp lemon juice and 2 tsp olive oil.

Dinner

- ► 6 ounces grilled lamb chops
- ► 3 cups baby spinach sautéed with 1 tsp minced garlic in 2 tsp olive oil
- ► 1 cup cooked brown rice

DAY 12

Breakfast

- ▶ 1 whole wheat English muffin spread with ½ mashed avocado and a scrambled egg
- ▶ 1 sliced apple sprinkled with cinnamon

Lunch

- ▶ 1 cup turkey chili
- ▶ 1 whole grain roll or 1 slice of whole grain bread
- ▶ 2 cups mixed greens tossed with ½ cup mixed vegetables and drizzled with 2 tbsp oil and vinegar dressing

Dinner

- ▶ 4 ounces grilled or broiled wild salmon brushed with 1 tsp olive oil
- ▶ 1 cup quinoa tossed with ¼ cup diced apples and 2 tbsp sunflower seeds
- ▶ 2 cups steamed or grilled asparagus sprinkled with 1 tbsp Parmesan cheese

DAY 13

Breakfast

- ▶ Omelet made with 2 whole eggs, ¼ cup sautéed spinach, ¼ cup diced red peppers, and 2 tbsp shredded aged cheddar cheese, cooked in 1 tsp olive oil

▶ 1 slice whole grain toast with trans-fat free margarine or butter

Lunch

▶ 1 whole wheat pita pocket filled with ½ cup chopped seasoned grilled chicken, ⅓ cup roasted peppers, and 1 cup mixed field greens, drizzled with 1 tbsp of olive oil and balsamic vinegar

Dinner

▶ 4 ounces grilled or broiled filet mignon
▶ 1 cup cooked wild rice
▶ 1½ cups mixed roasted vegetables tossed with 1 tbsp olive oil

DAY 14

Breakfast

▶ 1 yogurt parfait: 6 ounces plain yogurt, 1 sliced banana, 2 tbsp sunflower seeds, a pinch of cinnamon, ¼ cup uncooked rolled oats, and a splash of unsweetened almond milk

Lunch

▶ 1 grilled cheese sandwich: 2 slices whole grain bread, 1 slice of aged Swiss cheese, 2 slices tomato, and ½ cup baby spinach

- 1 cup roasted red pepper and tomato soup (or other vegetable or vegetable-bean soup)

Dinner

- 1, 4-ounce broiled chicken breast seasoned with lemon, garlic, and paprika, topped with 1 tbsp salsa and a squeeze of fresh lemon or lime
- 1½ cups grilled or roasted mixed vegetables (onions, peppers, zucchini, mushrooms, etc.)
- 1 cup cooked brown rice

Snack Ideas

- 22 almonds
- 4 walnut halves and 4 dried apricot halves
- 1 cup cubed cantaloupe topped with ½ cup plain yogurt and cinnamon
- 3 cups popcorn tossed with 1 tsp olive oil, 1 tbsp sunflower seeds, and ¼ tsp chili powder
- 1 whole grain crispbread cracker topped with ¼ avocado and 1 slice tomato
- 1 ounce aged cheddar cheese and ½ pear
- 1 whole grain crispbread topped with 1 tbsp almond butter, ¼ cup berries, and cinnamon
- ½ cup unsweetened applesauce, sprinkled with 1 tbsp crushed walnuts and a pinch cinnamon
- 1 slice whole grain toast topped with 1 tbsp peanut butter and ¼ banana

- ½ cup pineapple (fresh or canned in own juice) with a dollop of plain yogurt, sprinkled with 1 tsp chopped cashews
- 1 cup mixed berries topped with 1 tbsp sliced or slivered almonds
- ¾ cup plain yogurt with ½ cup blueberries and 1 tbsp chopped walnuts
- ½ avocado with 1 tbsp salsa and a squeeze of fresh lemon or lime
- 1 ounce of aged cheddar cheese and 14 almonds
- 10 cashews and an apple

By the end of this diet, you'll have learned what it feels like for your body to work optimally, and once you have reintroduced other foods (slowly and one at a time, documenting side effects!), you'll be aware of which foods you can enjoy occasionally and which are just too much for your system. You will most certainly be able to celebrate with a glass of wine and partake in birthday cake—remember, balance and moderation are the keys to healthy maintenance, not restriction!

The Paleo Plus Plan

■

If you got mostly A's on the Diagnostic Nutrition Test, the Paleo Plus Plan is your second of two diet options (the No-More-Back-Pain Meal Plan was the first). This plan reduces processed foods in general; eliminates dairy, alcohol, caffeine, and gluten; and minimizes the amounts of grains and beans to be eaten each day. It balances protein, high fiber sources of carbohydrate, and healthful sources of fat in each meal and snack. You'll enjoy whole grains and whole grain products, beans and lentils, and starchy vegetables such as sweet potatoes, corn, peas, potatoes, and winter squash, as well as nuts and nut butters and a little chocolate! This plan is a bit more regimented and recipe-oriented than the No-More-Back-Pain Meal Plan, but that might be helpful to you as you get on board with this new lifestyle!

PALEO PLUS SHOPPING LIST

Here is your grocery list with quantities! Stock your fridge with these whole foods and see what delicious meals and snacks you can create from these gut-friendly items in the "Recipes" section that follows.

PRODUCE

Large red onion (1 onion, about 1½ cups chopped)
Medium yellow onion (1 onion, about ¾ cup chopped)
Kale (1 bunch)

Sweet potato (4 medium)

Carrots (4 large)

Cremini mushrooms (1 cup chopped)

Cauliflower (6 cups chopped, 2 heads)

Broccoli (2 cups chopped)

Butter lettuce leaves (4 leaves)

Arugula (3 cups)

Spaghetti squash (1 small, about 1 pound)

Grape tomatoes (2 cups)

Pears (3)

Strawberries (¾ cup sliced)

Apples (3)

Blueberries (1 cup)

Bananas (3)

Grapes (at least 1 cup)

Garlic cloves (4)

Organic lemon (1, including the peel)

Zucchini (2)

Avocado (1)

Fresh basil (1 tablespoon)

REFRIGERATED/DAIRY/MEAT/POULTRY/FISH

Eggs (8 large)

Bone-in, skin-on chicken thighs (2, 6-ounce thighs)

Unsweetened almond milk (4 cups)

Wild salmon (2, 6-ounce filets)

Ground grass-fed beef (or bison) (8 ounces)

Peeled and cleaned raw shrimp (6 ounces)

Fresh salsa (¼ cup)

NON-PERISHABLES

Full-fat coconut milk (13.5-ounce can)

Almond butter (½ cup)

Pumpkin seeds (1 cup)

Chia seeds (¼ cup)

Walnuts (½ cup halves and pieces)

Quinoa (1⅓ cups)

Rolled oats (⅓ cup)

Brown rice (1¼ cups)

Unsalted chicken or beef bone broth (5 cups)

No-sugar-added marinara sauce (2 cups)

Dark chocolate (chips or bar, at least 65% cacao)
    (2½ ounces)

Unsweetened cocoa powder (1 tablespoon)

Organic sea salt potato chips (only ingredients
    potatoes, sea salt, oil) (2 ounces)

Navitas Naturals Maca Cashews (2 ounces) OR 22 dark
    chocolate–covered almonds

PANTRY ITEMS
(YOU MAY ALREADY HAVE SOME OF THESE)

Olive oil (¾ cup)

Coconut oil (4 teaspoons)

Balsamic vinegar (3 tablespoons)

Dried oregano (1½ teaspoons)

Sea salt

Black pepper

Garlic powder

Curry powder (2 teaspoons)

Turmeric powder (¼ teaspoon)

Ground cinnamon

Ground ginger

Paprika

Garbanzo beans (15-ounce can)

White beans (½ cup)

Mustard (½ teaspoon)

Vanilla extract (½ teaspoon)

Apple cider vinegar (3 teaspoons)

THE PALEO PLUS MEAL PLAN
WITH RECIPES

Nutritionists Willow Jarosh and Stephanie Clarke have created a day-by-day meal plan. Don't like something? It's okay. You can create your own meal—just try to use the recommended ingredients found on your shopping list so that you stick with the gist of the plan and keep fueling your body with these recommended types of foods. When in doubt, baked fish or meat, roast veggies, and a serving of quinoa or sweet potatoes will allow you to follow this plan. Remember, the goal is not to force feed yourself things you don't enjoy but rather to track your body responses and identify your triggers. Note any substitutions in your Symptom Journal in Chapter 7 so that you can see where your meal plan—and potentially your body reactions—diverge.

RECIPES FOR SEVEN DAYS OF PALEO PLUS MEALS AND SNACKS

These easy-to-follow recipes will keep you on track for the Paleo Plus Diet.

DAY 1

Breakfast

Egg and Kale Scramble

INGREDIENTS:
2 eggs
2 tsp olive oil
¼ cup red onion, sliced
½ cup chopped kale
apple, sliced

PREPARATION: Whisk together the eggs and set aside. Heat the olive oil in a medium skillet over medium heat. Add the sliced red onion, and sauté until soft, about five minutes. Add the chopped kale, and sauté until wilted, about three more minutes. Add the whisked eggs and cook, stirring occasionally, until firm, about three minutes. Serve with a sliced apple on the side.

Lunch

Veggie-Packed Bone Broth

INGREDIENTS:

3 cups unsalted chicken or beef bone broth

1 medium sweet potato, diced

½ cup carrot, diced

⅓ cup cremini mushrooms, chopped

½ cup broccoli florets

PREPARATION: Combine the chicken or beef broth with the sweet potato and carrot in a saucepan, and bring to a boil. Turn down to a simmer, cover, and cook until sweet potato is soft, about twenty minutes. Add the mushrooms and broccoli florets, cover, and simmer until broccoli is tender, about ten more minutes. Add salt to taste.

Dinner

Balsamic & Herb-Roasted Chicken with Quinoa and Cauliflower

INGREDIENTS:

1 tbsp balsamic vinegar

3 tsp olive oil

1 tsp dried oregano

½ tsp sea salt

¼ tsp black pepper

½ tsp garlic powder

(recipe continues)

2, 6-ounce, bone-in, skin-on chicken thighs
2 cups cauliflower, chopped
1¼ cups + 2 tbsp quinoa
1⅔ cups water

PREPARATION: Preheat oven to 425 degrees F. Whisk together the balsamic vinegar, one teaspoon of the olive oil, oregano, sea salt, black pepper, and garlic powder. Pour mixture over the two chicken thighs, and turn to coat.

Line a baking dish with parchment paper, and place chicken thighs inside. Bake until chicken reaches an internal temperature of 165 degrees F, about twenty-five minutes. Toss the cauliflower (florets and stems) with 2 teaspoons of the olive oil and a pinch of sea salt and black pepper. Spread cauliflower out on a baking sheet rubbed lightly with olive oil. Bake the cauliflower, stirring every ten minutes, until it's golden and soft, about twenty minutes. While the chicken and cauliflower bake, bring the quinoa to a boil in a small saucepan. Turn down to a simmer, cover, and cook until all water is absorbed, about twenty minutes.

Serve one cup of the cooked quinoa topped with a chicken thigh and the cauliflower. Freeze the remaining chicken thigh for dinner on Day 7. From the remaining quinoa, refrigerate one cup for breakfast on Day 2, and freeze one cup for dinner on Day 5.

Snack

Pear with Almond Butter

Slice a pear in half, and remove the seeds and stem. Spread 1 ½ teaspoons of almond butter on each half.

Treat

Dark Chocolate-Coconut Vegan Truffle

Chop up 2½ ounces of dark chocolate (or use chocolate chips so you don't need to chop up a bar), and combine with 2 tablespoons full-fat, canned coconut milk. Microwave for ten seconds, stir, and then microwave in five-second increments until the chocolate begins to soften, about fifteen more seconds, depending on your microwave. Stir until smooth, and refrigerate until firm, about forty-five minutes. Scoop mixture out with a spoon and roll into three equal balls. Roll each in enough cocoa powder to coat (about 1 tablespoon cocoa powder total). Eat one truffle now, and refrigerate the other two for Days 4 and 7.

DAY 2

Breakfast

Strawberry-Walnut Quinoa Cereal

INGREDIENTS:
1 cup quinoa, leftover
¼ cup canned coconut milk
¼ cup unsweetened almond milk
½ cup strawberries, sliced
1 tbsp walnuts, chopped

PREPARATION: Combine the leftover quinoa from Day 1 dinner with the canned coconut milk and unsweetened almond milk. Microwave just until heated, about thirty seconds. Top with the strawberries and walnuts.

Lunch

Loaded Tuna Salad

INGREDIENTS:
2 tsp olive oil
2 tsp apple cider vinegar
⅛ tsp sea salt
½ teaspoon mustard
pinch of black pepper
pinch of paprika
1 cup shredded carrot
½ cup chopped apple
1 tbsp chopped red onion

1, 5-ounce can of oil-packed albacore tuna

2 tbsp walnuts, chopped

PREPARATION: Whisk together the olive oil, apple cider vinegar, sea salt, mustard, and a pinch of black pepper and paprika. Toss together the carrot, apple, red onion, and the dressing. Top with the tuna and walnuts.

Dinner

Cauliflower-Garbanzo Curry Bowl

INGREDIENTS:

1¼ cups brown rice

2½ cups water

1 cup red onion, sliced

1 tbsp olive oil

2 tsp curry powder

¼ tsp sea salt

2 cups unsalted bone broth

4 cups cauliflower, roughly chopped

¼ cup canned coconut milk

1½ cups canned garbanzo beans

PREPARATION: Combine the brown rice and water in a saucepan, and bring to a boil. Turn down to a simmer, cover, and cook until all water is absorbed, about thirty minutes. While the rice cooks, sauté the red onion in olive oil in a large skillet over medium high heat, about seven minutes. Once the onions are soft, add the curry powder, sea salt, and bone broth.

(recipe continues)

Stir in the cauliflower, and allow to simmer until cauliflower begins to soften, about ten minutes. Add the coconut milk and garbanzo beans. Simmer until the liquid has decreased by one-third and the cauliflower begins to break apart, about ten more minutes.

Serve half of the cauliflower mixture over one cup of the cooked rice. Place the other half of the cauliflower mixture over one cup of rice in a container to refrigerate for lunch on Day 3. Store the remaining half-cup of rice in the freezer for lunch on Day 6.

Snack

Apple Slices with Cinnamon Almond Butter

Stir ½ teaspoon water and a pinch of ground cinnamon into 1 tablespoon of almond butter. Dip slices from one apple into the mixture.

Treat

Potato Chips

Enjoy 1 ounce (about 13 chips) organic sea salt potato chips (the only ingredients should be potatoes, sea salt, and oil).

DAY 3

Breakfast

Blue Magic Smoothie

INGREDIENTS:

1 cup blueberries

½ banana, ripe

¼ cup chopped carrot

¼ cup canned coconut milk

¼ tsp turmeric powder

¾ cup unsweetened almond milk

1 tbsp almond butter

PREPARATION: Combine the blueberries, banana, carrot, coconut milk, turmeric powder, almond milk, and almond butter in a blender. Blend until smooth. Add a handful of ice and blend again until frothy.

Lunch

Cauliflower-Garbanzo Curry Bowl (leftovers)

Have the leftover Cauliflower-Garbanzo Curry Bowl from dinner on Day 2.

Dinner

Walnut-Crusted Salmon with Broccoli

INGREDIENTS:

¼ cup walnuts

¼ tsp dried oregano

⅛ tsp sea salt

½ tsp mustard

2, 6-ounce wild salmon fillets

1½ cups broccoli florets, chopped

1 tbsp olive oil

½ clove garlic, chopped and crushed

1 tsp fresh lemon juice

¼ tsp lemon zest

PREPARATION: Preheat the oven to 425 degrees F. Combine the walnuts, oregano, and sea salt. Spread the mustard onto each of the salmon fillets, and press half of the walnut mixture onto the top of each. Place the salmon onto a parchment-paper-lined baking sheet, and bake until the fish flakes, about twenty minutes, checking at fifteen minutes.

While the fish cooks, sauté the broccoli florets and stems in the olive oil over medium heat until they begin soften, about twelve minutes. Add the garlic, and cook another minute. Remove from heat, and toss with the lemon juice and zest. Serve one salmon fillet with all of the broccoli. Refrigerate the other salmon fillet for lunch on Day 4.

Prep Ahead

Roasted Sea Salt Sweet Potatoes

2 medium sweet potatoes, about 3 cups diced

4 tsp coconut oil

½ tsp sea salt

While the oven is on, let's prepare sweet potatoes in advance for future meals. Dice the sweet potatoes, and toss with the coconut oil and sea salt. Place on a baking sheet in the oven until potato is soft and golden, about thirty minutes, stirring every fifteen minutes. You can cook these at the same time as the salmon.

Refrigerate the roasted sweet potato for lunch on Day 4, dinner on Day 6, and lunch on Day 7.

Prep Ahead

Chia Pudding

¼ cup chia seeds

1½ cups unsweetened almond milk

½ teaspoon vanilla extract

Combine the chia seeds with the almond milk and vanilla extract. Cover and refrigerate. This will be breakfast tomorrow!

Snack

Zucchini Salad with Walnuts

Combine ½ cup thinly sliced zucchini rounds with 1 teaspoon olive oil, 1 teaspoon apple cider vinegar, ¼ teaspoon lemon juice, and a pinch of sea salt and black pepper. Serve with 2 tablespoons walnuts.

Treat

Maca Cashews *or* Chocolate-Covered Almonds

Eat 1 ounce of Navitas Naturals brand Maca Cashews, OR have 11 (dark) chocolate-covered almonds.

DAY 4

Breakfast

Strawberry-Banana Chia Pudding

Pour half of the chia pudding mixture you made last night into a bowl. Stir in one mashed banana and 1 tablespoon almond butter. Top with ¼ cup sliced strawberries.

Lunch

Chopped Kale, Sweet Potato, and Salmon Salad

INGREDIENTS:

2 cups kale, chopped

1½ tsp olive oil

1½ tsp lemon juice

¼ tsp lemon zest

⅛ tsp sea salt

PREPARATION: Combine the kale with the olive oil, lemon juice and zest, and the sea salt. Using your hands, massage the dressing into the kale until the kale softens, about one minute. Add half of the leftover roasted sweet potato from Day 3 (about 1 cup), and toss lightly. Top with the leftover salmon from dinner on Day 3.

Dinner

Spaghetti Squash with Beef Marinara Sauce

INGREDIENTS:

1 lb spaghetti squash

½ cup yellow onion, chopped

1 tbsp olive oil

¼ tsp sea salt

1 clove garlic, chopped and crushed

¼ tsp dried oregano

⅛ tsp black pepper

8 ounces grass-fed ground beef or ground bison

2 cups no-sugar-added marinara sauce

(recipe continues)

Preparation: Preheat oven to 400 degrees F. Cut the spaghetti squash in half from end to end. Scoop out the seeds with a spoon, and place the squash, cut side down, in a baking dish with at least one-inch sides large enough to fit both squash halves. Pour water into the baking dish, so that it's about ⅛-inch deep. Bake until the squash is tender, about forty minutes.

While the squash cooks, sauté the onion in olive oil until tender, about five minutes. Add the sea salt, garlic, oregano, black pepper, and the beef. Cook until the ground beef is lightly browned, stirring to break up any chunks, about five minutes. Add the marinara sauce, and continue to simmer until the mixture thickens, about five more minutes.

Using a fork, scrape the squash flesh from the skin to form long strings. Place half of the squash onto a plate and top with half of the ground beef sauce. Place the other half of the squash and sauce in a container, and refrigerate for lunch on Day 5.

Prep Ahead

Remove quinoa from the freezer to use for dinner on Day 5.

Snack

Grape Tomatoes and Pumpkin Seeds

Eat 1 cup grape tomatoes with ¼ cup pumpkin seeds.

Treat

Hot Chocolate

Heat ½ cup of unsweetened almond milk until steaming hot. Pour into a mug with one of the chocolate truffles made on Day 1. Stir to dissolve.

DAY 5

Breakfast

Avocado Sweet Potato Toast

INGREDIENTS:
4, ⅛-inch-thick slices of sweet potato
½ avocado
½ tsp lemon juice
pinch of black pepper
2 tbsp pumpkin seeds
sea salt to taste

PREPARATION: Slice the sweet potato, and place in the toaster. Toast until soft and golden, about four toasting cycles. Mash the avocado with lemon juice and black pepper. Spread one-quarter of the avocado mixture onto each of the slices of sweet potato. Sprinkle the tops with the sea salt and pumpkin seeds. Spread lemon juice over the cut surface of the remaining avocado, cover with plastic wrap, and refrigerate.

Lunch

Spaghetti Squash with Beef Marinara (leftovers)

Eat the leftover spaghetti squash with beef marinara from dinner on Day 4.

Dinner

Garlic-Basil Shrimp with Grape Tomatoes and Carrot Fries

INGREDIENTS:

2 large carrots

2 tsp olive oil

pinch of sea salt

pinch of black pepper

1 tbsp olive oil

6 ounces shrimp

¾ cup grape tomatoes, halved

1 clove of garlic, crushed and chopped

1 tbsp sliced fresh basil

2 tbsp balsamic vinegar

leftover quinoa, thawed

PREPARATION: Preheat oven to 425 degrees F. Slice the carrots in half width-wise, and then slice each half in half lengthwise. Slice each quarter into 3–4 long sticks. Toss with 2 teaspoons of the olive oil and a pinch of sea salt and black pepper. Place in a single layer on a baking sheet, and bake until tender and golden, about fifteen to twenty minutes. Heat 1 tablespoon of the olive oil over medium-high heat. Add the shrimp, and cook until they just start to turn opaque, about three to four minutes, flipping shrimp halfway through to brown evenly on both sides. Add the grape tomatoes, garlic, basil, and balsamic vinegar, stirring ingredients to release any browned bits from the bottom.

Cook until shrimp is firm and completely opaque, about another minute. Remove shrimp from the pan, and add the thawed quinoa. Heat on low until warmed through. Serve shrimp over quinoa with half the carrot fries on the side.

Refrigerate the remaining half of the carrot fries for dinner on Day 6.

Prep Ahead

Pear-Almond Butter Overnight Oats

½ banana
2 tsp almond butter
pinch ground ginger
¾ cup unsweetened almond milk
⅓ cup rolled oats

Prepare overnight oats for Day 6 breakfast: mash half the banana and combine in a jar with the almond butter, ginger, almond milk, and rolled oats; stir to combine. Refrigerate overnight.

Prep Ahead

Hard-boil three eggs for lunch on Day 6 (for use in *Carrot-Pumpkin-Seed Egg Salad Lettuce Cups*).

Snack

Pear-Chia Pudding

Pour half the remaining chia pudding from breakfast on Day 4 into a bowl, and top with ¼ cup chopped pear.

Treat

Maca Cashews *or* Chocolate-Covered Almonds

Eat 1 ounce of Navitas Naturals brand Maca Cashews, OR have 11 (dark) chocolate-covered almonds.

DAY 6

Breakfast

Pear-Almond Butter Overnight Oats

Top the overnight oats made last night with half a pear, diced, and 2 teaspoons almond butter drizzled over the top.

Lunch

Carrot-Pumpkin-Seed Egg Salad Lettuce Cups

INGREDIENTS:
2 hard-boiled eggs and one hard-boiled egg white
2 tsp olive oil
⅛ tsp sea salt
⅛ tsp paprika

pinch of black pepper

1 tbsp chopped red onion

⅓ cup carrot, finely diced

3 tbsp pumpkin seeds

½ cup brown rice, leftover

4 butter lettuce leaves

PREPARATION: Mash all of the eggs with the olive oil, sea salt, paprika, and a pinch of black pepper. Stir in the onion, carrot, pumpkin seeds, and the half-cup brown rice saved from dinner on Day 2. Place mixture into the lettuce leaves, and eat like a burrito/wrap.

Dinner

Roasted Carrot, Arugula, and Mushroom Omelet

INGREDIENTS:

3 tsp olive oil

¼ cup yellow onion, chopped

½ cup cremini mushrooms

leftover carrot fries

1 cup arugula

⅛ tsp sea salt

2 eggs

1 tbsp unsweetened almond milk

1 cup leftover sweet potato

(recipe continues)

PREPARATION: Heat the olive oil in a medium skillet over medium heat. Add the onion and mushrooms, and cook until soft, about six minutes. Chop the leftover carrot fries from dinner on Day 5, and add to the pan, along with the and sea salt. Cook until arugula is wilted and carrots are heated through, about four more minutes. Remove from pan and set aside.

Whisk the eggs and almond milk in a bowl. Add another teaspoon olive oil to the pan in which you cooked the veggies, and heat over medium heat. Add the egg mixture, and cook until firm, gently scraping in the edges for even cooking. Add the veggie mixture to one half of pan, and fold the egg round in half to form an omelet. In the same skillet, heat half the leftover sweet potato (about one cup) until warmed through, and serve with the omelet.

Prep Ahead

Thaw the chicken from Day 1 to use for dinner tomorrow.

Snack

Almond Butter and Walnut Banana Slices

Slice half a banana into four rounds. Top each round with ½ teaspoon almond butter, and then press each into 1 teaspoon of crushed walnuts.

Treat

Potato Chips

Enjoy 1 ounce (about 13 chips) organic sea salt potato chips (the only ingredients should be potatoes, sea salt, and oil).

DAY 7

Breakfast

Avocado Baked Egg with Salsa

INGREDIENTS:
½ avocado
¼ cup salsa
1 egg
sea salt and pepper to taste
½ pear
1 tbsp almond butter

PREPARATION: Preheat oven to 350 degrees F. Scoop out enough of the avocado flesh around where the pit was to allow an egg white and yolk to fit. Combine any avocado you scoop out with the salsa, and set aside. Crack the egg into the center of the avocado half, and sprinkle with salt and pepper. Bake at 350 until the egg is firm, about fifteen minutes. Top with the salsa-avocado mixture, and serve with the pear spread with almond butter on the side.

Lunch

Sweet Potato and White Bean Salad

INGREDIENTS:
2 tsp olive oil
2 tsp lemon juice
¼ tsp lemon zest
⅛ tsp sea salt
pinch of black pepper
pinch of paprika
½ cup canned white beans, rinsed and drained
2 cups arugula
1 cup leftover roasted sweet potatoes
1 tbsp walnuts, chopped

PREPARATION: Whisk together the olive oil, lemon juice and zest, sea salt, and a pinch each of black pepper and paprika. Set aside. Toss together the beans with the arugula, the final cup of leftover roasted sweet potatoes, and chopped walnuts. Add the lemon and oil dressing, and toss to coat.

Dinner

Zoodles with Garlic-Almond Butter Sauce

INGREDIENTS:
1 medium zucchini or 1½ cups zucchini noodles
1 tbsp olive oil
1 cup grape tomatoes
⅛ tsp salt

1½ tbsp almond butter

2 tsp apple cider vinegar

1 tsp water

1 clove of garlic, crushed and diced

PREPARATION: To get the zucchini "noodles," use a julienne peeler or a spiralizer to create strands from the zucchini. In a medium skillet, heat the olive oil over medium-high heat. Add the zucchini noodles and cook, stirring often, until they begin to soften, about eight minutes. Add the tomatoes, salt, and pepper. Continue to cook until tomatoes crack open, about five more minutes. Chop the leftover chicken, and add to the pan, stirring to combine. Heat on low until the chicken is warmed through. Stir together the almond butter, apple cider vinegar, garlic, sea salt, and 1 teaspoon water. Pour the almond butter mixture over the zucchini mixture, and toss to coat.

Snack

Apple-Cinnamon Chia Pudding

Stir ⅛ teaspoon ground cinnamon into the remaining chia pudding and top with ¼ cup chopped apple.

Treat

Dark Chocolate-Coconut Truffle

Eat the last truffle!

PALEO PLUS BONUS DAYS

DAY 1

Breakfast

Raspberry Almond Butter Sweet Potato Toast

INGREDIENTS:
4, ⅛-inch-thick slices sweet potato
2 tbsp almond butter
½ cup halved raspberries
cinnamon (optional)

PREPARATION: Place the sweet potato slices in the toaster and toast until soft and golden, about four toasting cycles. Spread each slice with ½ tablespoon almond butter and 2 tablespoons raspberries. Add cinnamon if desired.

Lunch

Mediterranean Quinoa Salad Bowl with Chicken

INGREDIENTS:
½ cup cooked quinoa
¼ cup rinsed and drained canned chickpeas
3 ounces boneless grilled chicken
½ cup chopped roasted peppers
2 tbsp chopped parsley
2 tbsp olive oil
1 tsp lemon juice

1 tsp white wine vinegar

⅛ tsp salt

⅛ tsp cumin

dash of cayenne pepper

PREPARATION: Toss quinoa with chickpeas, roasted peppers, and chopped parsley. Dress with olive oil whisked with lemon juice, white wine vinegar, salt, cumin, and dash of cayenne pepper.

Dinner

Grass-Fed Beef Burger and Salad

INGREDIENTS:

⅛ tsp salt

2 tsp balsamic vinegar, divided

pinch ground black pepper

4 ounces grass-fed ground beef

2 tsp olive oil

1 medium baked potato, sliced in half lengthwise

1 tbsp hummus

1 slice tomato

1 cup roughly chopped romaine lettuce

½ cup diced carrot

½ cup diced cucumber

PREPARATION: Add balsamic vinegar, salt, and black pepper to a mixing bowl. Stir in beef and mix until spices are evenly distributed. Form into a patty about ¼ inch thick. Heat a

(recipe continues)

skillet over medium-high heat. Add 1 teaspoon olive oil and place patty into the pan. Cook until desired doneness, flipping once. About three minutes on each side will yield medium. Place the burger on the potato, spread with hummus and top with lettuce and tomato. Serve with a salad made from chopped romaine lettuce, diced carrot, diced cucumber, 1 teaspoon olive oil, 1 teaspoon balsamic vinegar, and a pinch of salt and pepper all tossed together.

DAY 2

Breakfast

Red Pepper Omelet

INGREDIENTS:
2 tsp olive oil, divided
½ cup chopped red bell peppers
2 eggs
1 egg white
1 apple, sliced
pinch of cinnamon

PREPARATION: In a small skillet over medium high heat, sauté peppers in olive oil until soft, about five minutes. Remove from skillet and set aside.

Turn heat down to medium, add 1 teaspoon olive oil to the skillet. Whisk eggs and egg white together with a splash of water and pour into skillet. Cook eggs for three–four minutes until set and firm on the bottom. Add peppers to the top of the egg. Fold one side of the omelet over the top of the other. Cook until the egg middles are no longer runny, about two more minutes.

Serve omelet with apple slices dusted with a pinch of cinnamon.

Lunch

Egg Salad with Grapes, Avocado, and Walnuts

INGREDIENTS:
2 hard-boiled eggs
1 tbsp regular mayonnaise
1 tsp lemon juice
¼ cup chopped celery
black pepper to taste
½ avocado, sliced
2 cups baby spinach
1 cup grapes
2 tbsp crushed walnuts

PREPARATION: Lightly mash hard-boiled eggs and stir in mayonnaise and lemon juice. Add chopped celery and black pepper. Place egg salad on baby spinach leaves and top with avocado, half the grapes, and walnuts. Serve with the remaining half of grapes on the side.

Dinner

Grilled Lamb Chops, Sweet Potato Fries, and Broccoli

INGREDIENTS:

1, 4-ounce lamb chop

½ medium sweet potato

3 tsp olive oil, divided

¼ tsp salt

¼ tsp cumin

⅛ tsp cinnamon

⅛ tsp black pepper

2 cups broccoli florets

2 tsp lemon juice

¼ tsp lemon zest

1 tsp olive oil

PREPARATION: Pre-heat oven to 400 degrees F. Chop the sweet potato into fry-shaped pieces. Toss sweet potatoes with 2 teaspoons olive oil and arrange evenly on a baking sheet. Bake until crisp, about twenty minutes, turning halfway through cooking time.

While sweet potatoes cook, pat lamb dry with paper towels (this helps produce a nice golden crust as it cooks). Rub both sides with the blend of salt, pepper, cumin, and cinnamon. Heat a grill or grill pan over medium high heat. Grill lamb chops about four–five minutes per side or until cooked to 145 degrees F for medium rare.

Steam broccoli florets and toss with lemon juice, lemon zest, and 1 teaspoon olive oil. Serve lamb chops with fries and broccoli.

DAY 3

Breakfast

Strawberry-Walnut Chia Pudding

INGREDIENTS:

3 tbsp chia seeds

1 cup unsweetened vanilla almond milk

¼ ripe banana, mashed

⅛ tsp cinnamon

¾ cup sliced or chopped strawberries

1 tbsp chopped walnuts

PREPARATION: Whisk chia seeds with almond milk, banana, and cinnamon. Let the mixture sit, covered, in the fridge for at least two hours or overnight.

Top with chopped walnuts, strawberries, and a sprinkle of cinnamon, if desired.

Lunch

Salmon and Quinoa with Peanut Sauce

INGREDIENTS:

1 tbsp peanut butter

¾ tsp tamari (or soy sauce)

¼ tsp fresh or dried ginger

2 tsp rice vinegar

2 tsp water

1 cup cooked quinoa

4 ounces roasted wild salmon (or chicken breast)

(recipe continues)

½ cup shredded carrot

½ cup chopped baby spinach

PREPARATION: Whisk together peanut butter, tamari (or soy sauce), ginger, rice vinegar, and water. Toss shredded carrot and spinach with quinoa. Top with salmon and drizzle with peanut sauce.

Dinner

Grilled Chicken Lettuce Wraps with Chipotle Cabbage Slaw

INGREDIENTS:

2 tsp mayonnaise

2 tsp lime juice

¼ tsp chipotle pepper powder

1 cup shredded purple cabbage

3 tbsp chopped cashews

4 ounces cooked shredded chicken breast

4 butter lettuce leaves

¼ of an avocado, cubed

fresh cilantro

PREPARATION: Whisk together mayonnaise, lime juice, chipotle pepper powder, and sea salt and toss with shredded purple cabbage and cashews. Top each lettuce leaf with ¼ of the chicken, ¼ of the slaw, 1 tablespoon of avocado, and fresh cilantro (if you like it!). Serve any slaw that wouldn't fit into the lettuce leaves on the side.

The Low FODMAPS Diet

◼

Some people experience sensitivity to certain types of carbohydrates. If your body isn't able to adequately digest these carbohydrates, they pass into the large intestine where they cause gas, bloating, and diarrhea or constipation. These specific types of carbohydrates are called FODMAPS, which stands for Fermentable Oligosaccharides, Disaccharides, Monosaccharides and Polyols. This plan removes all foods that contain FODMAPS.

It can help restore digestive balance and ensure that there aren't undigested foods reaching the large intestine to cause irritating or painful symptoms. Even without food containing these carbohydrates, the FODMAPS Plan still delivers a balance of nutrients for overall health and stable energy levels. You'll find foods such as gluten-free breads and corn tortillas so that you can have your comfort foods—such as French toast and tacos—without experiencing painful or uncomfortable side effects.

LOW FODMAP SHOPPING LIST

Here is your grocery list! Stock your fridge with these FODMAP-free foods, and see what delicious meals and snacks you can create in the "Recipes" section that follows.

PRODUCE

Japanese eggplant (3 small or 1 large eggplant)
Baby spinach

Carrots (1 lb, about 5 medium carrots)
Blueberries (2 cups / 1 pint)
Banana (1)
Avocado (2)
Grape tomatoes (1 pound)
Cucumber (2 medium)
Scallions (1 bunch)
Lemons (2)
Russet potatoes (3 large)
Yellow/golden potato (1 medium)
Green beans (1 ½ cups)
Red bell pepper (2)
Kiwi (1)
Grapefruit (2)
Grapes (at least 1 cup)
Basil (small bunch)
Parsley (small bunch)
Ginger (1 small piece)
Olives, black or Kalamata (Greek) (7)

REFRIGERATED/DAIRY/MEAT

Eggs (1 dozen large)
Ground beef (12 ounces, preferably grass-fed)
Skinless chicken breast (12 ounces)
Salmon (1, 4-ounce filet or steak)
Cheddar cheese (block form, 3 ounces)
Unsweetened almond milk (1⅔ cup)

NON-PERISHABLES

Can tuna packed in olive oil (1, 5-ounce can)
Almond butter (⅓ cup)

Dark chocolate (65% or higher cocoa, 2 ounces)
Corn chips (2 ounces; only ingredients should be corn,
    oil, and salt)
Whole almonds (14)
Sliced almonds (½ cup)
Sunflower seeds
Quinoa (1 ½ cups)
Brown rice (½ cup)
Brown rice bread (1 loaf)
Lower sodium soy sauce
Rice vinegar

FROZEN

Frozen pineapple (1 cup)
Fruit sorbet (1 cup)

PANTRY ITEMS
(you may already have some of these)

Olive oil
Balsamic vinegar
Maple syrup
Salt
Pepper
Ground turmeric
Ground cinnamon
Hot sauce (such as "Frank's")
Vanilla extract
Ketchup (with no high fructose corn syrup)
Brown sugar

RECIPES FOR SEVEN DAYS OF FODMAPS MEALS AND SNACKS

Nutritionists Willow Jarosh and Stephanie Clarke have created a day-by-day meal plan with easy-to-follow recipes that will help guide you through the FODMAPS plan. Don't like something? It's okay. You can create your own meal—just try to use the recommended ingredients found on your shopping list—or swap in other foods that will help you keep your diet free of FODMAPS this week!

DAY 1

Breakfast

Brown Rice French Toast with Blueberries

INGREDIENTS:
1 egg
2 tbsp unsweetened almond milk
⅛ tsp ground cinnamon
½ tsp vanilla extract
2 slices of brown rice bread
½ cup blueberries

PREPARATION: In a shallow bowl, whisk together the egg, almond milk, cinnamon, and vanilla extract. Dip two slices of brown rice bread in the egg mixture, letting each side of the bread soak in the egg for about one minute.

Heat a medium skillet over medium heat, and add the coconut oil. Add the egg-soaked bread slices to the skillet, and cook the French toast pieces about one-and-a-half to two minutes per side, or until golden brown. Top the French toast with the blueberries.

Lunch

Chopped Spinach Salad with Avocado and Tuna

INGREDIENTS:

2 cups baby spinach, chopped

¼ cup carrot, shredded

½ cup cucumber, chopped

½ cup tomato, chopped

2 tbsp avocado, cubed

1, 5-ounce can tuna packed in olive oil, drained

1 tbsp lemon juice

2 tsp olive oil

garlic powder to taste

black pepper to taste

PREPARATION: Combine the spinach with the carrot, cucumber, tomato, avocado, and canned tuna. Drizzle with the lemon juice, olive oil, and add garlic powder and black pepper to taste.

Dinner

Grass-Fed Beef Burger with Baked Fries and Sautéed Spinach

NOTE: *You'll use one burger for dinner tonight, refrigerate one for lunch on Day 2, and freeze one for Day 6. You'll also save one-third of the fries you make tonight to use tomorrow at breakfast.*

(recipe continues)

INGREDIENTS:

1 large Russet potato

3 tsp olive oil

dash of salt

dash of paprika

12 ounces grass-fed ground beef

½ cup carrots, finely grated

1 tbsp parsley

1 tbsp chopped green onion (green parts only)

¼ tsp black pepper

¼ tsp salt

3 cups baby spinach

PREPARATION: Preheat oven to 420 degrees F. Wash and chop the potato into fry-shaped pieces. Toss the fries in 2 teaspoons of the olive oil and sprinkle salt and paprika. Layer the fries evenly on a baking sheet lined with parchment or foil. Bake until potatoes are tender and golden on the edges, turning once throughout cooking time, about fifteen to twenty minutes. Reserve two-thirds of the fries for dinner tonight. Refrigerate the remaining third to use in tomorrow's breakfast scramble.

While the fries bake, combine the beef with the carrots, parsley, green onion, pepper, and salt. Form into three even patties. Heat one teaspoon of the olive oil in a medium-to-large skillet over medium-high heat. Once oil is hot, add burgers, and cook until cooked through, about three to four minutes per side.

Sauté the spinach in the remaining teaspoon olive oil until wilted. Serve over the burger and alongside the fries. Serve with ketchup on the side for dipping.

Snack

Bell Pepper and Olives

½ cup sliced red bell pepper with 6 olives

Treat

Corn Chips

1 ounce corn chips (only ingredients should be corn, oil, and salt)

DAY 2

Breakfast

Potato Egg Scramble

INGREDIENTS:
1 egg + 2 egg whites
1 tsp oil
½ cup baby spinach, chopped
black pepper, if desired
leftover baked fries

PREPARATION: Whisk the eggs together with 1 tablespoon water. Add the spinach and pepper, if desired. Set aside.

Heat a medium skillet over medium-low heat. Add the olive oil, and heat one minute. Cut the leftover baked fries into ¼-inch pieces, and add the pieces to the skillet, cooking for one minute to warm. Add the egg mixture and cook, scrambling eggs, until they are cooked through, about two minutes. Serve scramble with hot sauce, if desired.

Lunch

Beef Tacos

INGREDIENTS:
leftover beef burger, chopped or crumbled
dash of chili powder
dash of cumin
2 small corn tortillas
½ cup chopped tomato
½ cup shredded carrot
1 tbsp diced avocado

PREPARATION: Chop or crumble leftover burger, toss with a dash of chili powder and cumin, and heat until warm. Add beef to two small corn tortillas, and top each with the tomato, carrot, and avocado.

Dinner

Quinoa and Spinach Salad with Lemon Turmeric Dressing

> **NOTE:** *the following meal makes two servings plus an extra serving of quinoa. Use one serving for dinner today, and store the other serving for lunch on Day 4. You'll use the remaining quinoa in tomorrow's lunch.*

INGREDIENTS:
2 cups cooked quinoa
¼ cup toasted sliced almonds
1½ cups baby spinach, chopped

1 cup chopped red bell pepper
2 tsp olive oil
2 tsp lemon juice
pinch of salt
pinch of chopped basil
pinch of ground turmeric

PREPARATION: Cook the quinoa according to package directions. Toss the cooked quinoa with the almonds, spinach, and bell pepper. Whisk together the olive oil, lemon juice, salt, basil, and turmeric. Divide quinoa salad in half, and toss one half with the lemon juice dressing. Store the undressed half for lunch on Day 4.

Snack

Kiwi and Almonds

Pair 1 kiwi with 14 almonds.

Treat

Broiled Grapefruit with Ginger Maple Syrup

Preheat broiler. Mix 2 teaspoons maple syrup with ½ teaspoon fresh chopped ginger (ginger optional). Cut a grapefruit in half, leaving the skin on. Then cut a small slice off of the round ends so the grapefruit halves sit upright. Brush maple syrup over the flesh of the grapefruit halves. Broil for three to four minutes, or until the top is uniform and bubbly.

DAY 3

Breakfast

Breakfast Tostada

INGREDIENTS:

1 egg
1 tsp olive oil
1 corn tortilla
2 tbsp smashed avocado
¼ cup chopped tomatoes
1 tbsp chopped olives

PREPARATION: Heat a medium skillet over medium high heat and fry the egg in 1 teaspoon of the olive oil. Remove egg from skillet and set aside on a plate. Heat the remaining ½ teaspoon olive oil in the skillet, and heat the tortilla until warmed through and slightly crisp on each side. Spread the avocado over the tortilla; then add egg, and top with the tomatoes and olives.

Lunch

Spinach, Quinoa, and Grapefruit Salad

INGREDIENTS:

2 cups baby spinach, chopped
½ cup of leftover quinoa
½ grapefruit, peeled and sliced into ½ rounds
2 tbsp toasted sunflower seeds
2 tsp olive oil
2 tsp balsamic vinegar
dash of salt and pepper

PREPARATION: Combine the spinach with the quinoa and top with the grapefruit and sunflower seeds. Dress with the olive oil whisked with the balsamic vinegar and a dash of salt and pepper.

Dinner

Chicken and Eggplant Stir-Fry

NOTE: *You'll cook two servings of the stir-fry plus an extra portion of chicken to freeze for Day 6.*

INGREDIENTS:

1 tbsp canola oil
1 tsp sesame oil
12 ounces (¾ pound) skinless, boneless chicken breast
salt and pepper to taste
2 small Japanese eggplants
1 cup cubed red bell pepper
¼ cup chicken broth
1½ tbsp low sodium soy sauce
1½ tbsp rice vinegar
1 tsp brown sugar
2 tsp fresh chopped ginger

PREPARATION: Heat a skillet over medium-high heat, and add the canola oil and sesame oil. Add the chicken breast sprinkled with salt and pepper, along with the eggplants and bell pepper. Stir-fry until chicken is browned and veggies are softened, about five to seven minutes.

(recipe continues)

Meanwhile, whisk together the chicken broth, soy sauce, rice vinegar, and brown sugar. Set aside. Add the ginger to the skillet, and sauté one minute longer, stirring to incorporate. Add the soy sauce mixture, scraping the bottom of the skillet to release any browned bits. Cook for another two to three minutes, until sauce is incorporated.

Separate one-quarter of the chicken, and freeze for use in lunch on Day 6. Divide the remaining stir fry into two portions, eating one for dinner and refrigerating the other for use in lunch on Day 5.

Snack

Cucumber Salad

Toss 1 cup cucumber slices with 1 teaspoon olive oil and 1 teaspoon balsamic vinegar. Add 1 tablespoon sliced almonds.

Treat

Fruit Sorbet

½ cup all-fruit sorbet (the only ingredients should be fruit)

DAY 4

Breakfast

Blueberry, Spinach, Almond Butter, and Almond Milk Smoothie

INGREDIENTS:

1 cup blueberries

1 cup baby spinach

¾ cup unsweetened almond milk

1 tbsp almond butter

1 cup ice

PREPARATION: Blend the blueberries, spinach, almond milk, almond butter, and ice in a blender until smooth.

Lunch

Leftover Spinach, Quinoa, and Grapefruit Salad

INGREDIENTS:

2 tsp olive oil

2 tsp lemon juice

1 tsp chopped basil

pinch of salt

pinch of ground turmeric

PREPARATION: Whisk together the olive oil, lemon juice, basil, and a pinch of salt and ground turmeric. Toss the leftover serving of quinoa salad from dinner on Day 2 with the dressing before serving.

Dinner

Baked Salmon with Lemon-Olive-Parsley Salsa, Baked Potato, and Green Beans

NOTE: *You'll cook two potatoes, one to use tonight and another to use on Day 5. And you'll reserve half the salmon for dinner on Day 5.*

INGREDIENTS:

2 Russet potatoes
1, 8-ounce fillet of salmon
2 tbsp chopped parsley
2 tbsp chopped black or Kalamata olives
2 tbsp lemon juice
3½ tsp olive oil
1 cup green beans

PREPARATION: Preheat oven to 425 degrees F. Pierce the potatoes in three to four places with the tines of a fork. Place potatoes on a foil-lined baking sheet in the oven, and bake until tender, about fifty minutes.

Top the non-skin side of the salmon with a mixture of the parsley, black or Kalamata olives, lemon juice, and olive oil. Toss the green beans in the olive oil, making sure they're evenly coated.

When the potatoes have been in the oven for about thirty minutes, add the green beans, evenly spaced, and the salmon to the baking sheet. Cook until the green beans are tender, the potato flesh is fork tender, and the salmon is cooked through and flakes with a fork, about fifteen to twenty minutes. Serve one-half of the salmon with the green beans and one of the baked potatoes. Refrigerate the remaining half of salmon for dinner on Day 5.

Snack

Grapefruit with Sunflower Seeds

1 grapefruit with 2 tablespoons sunflower seeds on the side

Treat

Dark Chocolate

1 ounce dark chocolate (preferably 70% cacao or higher)

DAY 5

Breakfast

Egg-Quinoa-Spinach Scramble

INGREDIENTS:
1 tsp olive oil
2 eggs
1 tbsp water
½ cup cooked quinoa (remaining from Day 2)
½ cup spinach, chopped

PREPARATION: Heat the olive oil in a medium skillet over medium heat. Add the eggs whisked with a tablespoon water, the spinach, and the quinoa (remaining from Day 2). Scramble until eggs are cooked through. Serve with hot sauce, if desired.

Lunch

Leftover Chicken Stir-Fry on a Baked Potato

Heat the leftover serving of chicken stir-fry from Day 3, and serve over the leftover baked potato from Day 4. Add hot sauce, if desired.

Dinner

> **NOTE:** *Defrost chicken in the refrigerator tonight so that it's thawed for lunch on Day 6.*

Salmon Tostadas

INGREDIENTS:

2 tsp olive oil

2 corn tortillas

2 tbsp smashed avocado

4 ounces flaked roasted salmon

1 tbsp chopped spinach

4 tablespoons chopped tomato

PREPARATION: Heat the olive oil in a medium skillet over medium-high heat. Place the corn tortillas in the skillet, and cook until slightly crispy, turning once. Place the avocado on each of the tortillas, and top each with the salmon, spinach, and tomato.

Snack

Avocado-Tomato-Cucumber Toast

Spread a slice of toasted brown rice bread with 1 tablespoon avocado, and layer with 6 cucumber slices and 2–3 sliced grape tomatoes. Add a dash of sea salt and black pepper, if desired.

Treat

Fruit Sorbet

½ cup all fruit sorbet
(the only ingredients should be fruit)

DAY 6

NOTE: *Defrost the leftover beef burger from dinner on Day 1 for dinner tonight.*

Breakfast

Almond Butter Banana Toast

INGREDIENTS:
1 slice brown rice bread, toasted
1½ tbsp almond butter
½ banana, sliced
cinnamon to taste

PREPARATION: Spread the toasted brown rice bread with the almond butter, and top with one-half of the banana and cinnamon to taste.

NOTE: *Freeze the other half of the banana in chunks to use for breakfast on Day 7.*

Lunch

Tomato-Cucumber Salad with Chicken and Avocado

INGREDIENTS:
1 cup cucumber, diced
1 cup halved grape tomatoes
2 tbsp cubed avocado
leftover chicken (Day 3)
1 tsp olive oil
1 tsp balsamic vinegar

PREPARATION: Toss the cucumber with the tomatoes, avocado, and leftover chicken. Dress with the olive oil and balsamic vinegar.

Dinner

Beef Burger, Green Beans, and Red Pepper Sauté

INGREDIENTS:
2 tsp olive oil
½ cup green beans, cut
½ cup sliced red bell pepper
dash of salt
dash of pepper
splash of lemon juice
1 cup cooked brown rice
leftover beef burger

PREPARATION: Heat a medium sauté pan over medium-high heat. Add one teaspoon of the olive oil, the green beans, and the bell pepper, and sauté until tender, about six minutes. Add a dash of salt and pepper and a splash of lemon juice. Serve vegetables with a side of the rice tossed with the remaining teaspoon olive oil and the heated leftover burger. Drizzle with hot sauce, if desired.

Snack

Hard-Boiled Egg and Carrot Sticks

Pair 1 hard-boiled egg with 1 cup carrot sticks.

Treat

Dark Chocolate

1 ounce dark chocolate (preferably 70% cacao or higher)

DAY 7

Breakfast

Pineapple-Banana-Carrot Smoothie

INGREDIENTS:
1 cup frozen pineapple
½ banana (frozen in chunks from Day 6)
½ cup carrot, grated or chopped
1¼ cups unsweetened almond milk
1 tbsp almond butter

(recipe continues)

PREPARATION: In a blender, combine the pineapple with the frozen half-banana from Day 6, carrot, almond milk, and almond butter. Blend until smooth.

Lunch

Bento "Box"

Gather 2 hard-boiled eggs, ½ cup blueberries, and ½ cup carrot and celery sticks dipped in 2 tablespoons almond butter.

Dinner

Spinach, Eggplant, and Potato Frittata with Carrot Fries

INGREDIENTS:
2 carrots
2½ tsp olive oil
pinch of salt
½ cup diced eggplant
½ cup diced white potato
½ cup baby spinach, chopped
2 whisked eggs

PREPARATION: Preheat the oven to 400 degrees F. Cut the carrots into fry-shape pieces, and toss with 1½ teaspoons of the olive oil and a pinch of salt. Then spread evenly on a foiled-lined baking sheet. Bake for fifteen to twenty minutes, turning halfway through cooking time, until carrots are lightly browned and crisp.

Meanwhile, heat a medium oven-safe skillet over medium heat. Add the remaining teaspoon olive oil, the eggplant, and the diced potato. Sauté until potatoes are soft, about seven minutes; then add the spinach to the skillet, and stir to combine. Add the eggs, and swirl to spread the eggs evenly throughout the skillet. Cook for two to three minutes or until eggs are firm on the bottom. Then place the skillet in the oven, and cook until eggs are cooked throughout, about five to seven more minutes. Serve frittata with carrot fries.

Snack

Grape Tomatoes, Cucumber, and Avocado

Pair ½ cup halved grape tomatoes with ½ cup chopped cucumber and 2 tablespoons diced avocado.

Treat

Corn Chips

1 ounce corn chips (only ingredients should be corn, oil, and salt)

LOW FODMAPS BONUS DAYS

DAY 1

Breakfast

Raspberry Almond Butter Toast

INGREDIENTS:
2 slices brown rice bread
2 tbsp almond butter
½ cup halved raspberries
cinnamon (optional)

PREPARATION: Spread each slice of toast with 1 tablespoon almond butter and ¼ cup sliced raspberries. Add cinnamon if desired.

Lunch

Mediterranean Quinoa Salad Bowl

INGREDIENTS:
1 cup cooked quinoa
⅓ cup crushed walnuts
½ cup chopped roasted peppers
2 tbsp chopped parsley
1 tbsp olive oil
1 tsp lemon juice
1 tsp white wine vinegar
1 tsp honey
⅛ tsp salt

⅛ tsp cumin

dash of cayenne pepper

PREPARATION: Toss quinoa with chickpeas, feta cheese, roasted peppers, and chopped parsley. Dress with olive oil whisked lemon juice, white wine vinegar, honey, salt, cumin, and dash of cayenne pepper.

Dinner

Grass-Fed Beef Burger and Salad

INGREDIENTS:

⅛ tsp salt

2 tsp balsamic vinegar, divided

pinch ground black pepper

4 ounces grass-fed ground beef

2 tsp olive oil, divided

1 gluten free hamburger bun

1 tbsp hummus

1 slice tomato

1 cup roughly chopped romaine lettuce

½ cup diced carrot

½ cup diced cucumber

PREPARATION: Add balsamic vinegar, salt, and black pepper to a mixing bowl. Stir in beef and mix until spices are evenly distributed. Form into a patty about ¼ inch thick. Heat a skillet over medium-high heat. Add 1 teaspoon olive oil and place patty into the pan. Cook until desired doneness, flipping once.

(recipe continues)

About 3 minutes on each side will yield medium. Place the burger on the bun spread with hummus and top with lettuce and tomato. Serve with a salad made from chopped romaine lettuce, diced carrot, diced cucumber, 1 teaspoon olive oil, 1 teaspoon balsamic vinegar, and a pinch of salt and pepper all tossed together.

DAY 2

Breakfast

Red Pepper Omelet

INGREDIENTS:
2 tsp olive oil, divided
½ cup chopped red bell peppers
2 eggs
1 egg white
1 slice brown rice toast
1 teaspoon olive oil

PREPARATION: In a small skillet over medium high heat, sauté peppers in olive oil until soft, about 5 minutes. Remove from skillet and set aside.

Turn heat down to medium, add 1 teaspoon olive oil to the skillet. Whisk eggs and egg white together with a splash of water and pour into skillet. Cook eggs for three–four minutes until set and firm on the bottom. Add peppers to the top of the egg. Fold one side of the omelet over the top of the other. Cook until the egg middles are no longer runny, about two more minutes.

Serve omelet with 1 slice brown rice toast with 1 teaspoon olive oil.

Lunch

Egg Salad Sandwich with Grapes

INGREDIENTS:
2 hard boiled eggs
1 tbsp regular mayonnaise
1 tsp lemon juice
¼ cup chopped celery
black pepper to taste
2 slices brown rice bread
½ cup baby spinach
1 cup grapes

PREPARATION: Mash hard boiled eggs and stir in mayonnaise and lemon juice. Add chopped celery and black pepper. Place egg salad on 1 slice of brown rice bread top with baby spinach leaves and the other slice of bread. Serve with 1 cup grapes.

Dinner

Grilled Lamb Chops, Sweet Potato Fries, and Broccoli

INGREDIENTS:

1, 4-ounce lamb chop

½ medium sweet potato

3 tsp olive oil, divided

¼ tsp salt

¼ tsp cumin

⅛ tsp cinnamon

⅛ tsp black pepper

1 cup broccoli florets

½ tsp lemon juice

⅛ tsp lemon zest

   (optional but recommended for lots of flavor)

PREPARATION: Pre-heat oven to 400 degrees F. Chop the sweet potato into fry-shaped pieces. Toss sweet potatoes with 2 teaspoons olive oil and arrange evenly on a baking sheet. Bake until crisp, about twenty minutes, turning halfway through cooking time.

While sweet potatoes cook, pat lamb dry with paper towels (this helps produce a nice golden crust as it cooks). Rub both sides with the blend of salt, pepper, cumin, and cinnamon. Heat a grill or grill pan over medium high heat. Grill lamb chops about four–five minutes per side or until cooked to 145 degrees F for medium rare.

Steam broccoli florets until crisp but tender and toss with lemon juice, lemon zest, and 1 teaspoon olive oil. Serve lamb chops with fries and broccoli.

DAY 3

Breakfast

Strawberry Chia Pudding with Brown Sugar

INGREDIENTS:
3 tbsp chia seeds
1 cup unsweetened vanilla almond milk
1 tsp brown sugar
⅛ tsp cinnamon
¾ cup sliced or chopped strawberry
1 tbsp chopped walnuts

PREPARATION: Whisk chia seeds with almond milk, brown sugar, and cinnamon. Let the mixture sit, covered, in the fridge for at least two hours or overnight.

Top with chopped walnuts, strawberries, and a sprinkle of cinnamon, if desired.

Lunch

Soba Noodle Salad with Salmon and Peanut Sauce

INGREDIENTS:
1 tbsp peanut butter
¾ tsp gluten free tamari (or soy sauce)
¼ tsp fresh ginger (or a pinch dried)
2 tsp rice vinegar
2 tsp water

(recipe continues)

1 cup cooked buckwheat (soba) noodles

1, 4-ounce roasted wild salmon (or chicken breast)

½ cup shredded carrot

½ cup chopped baby spinach

PREPARATION: Whisk together peanut butter, tamari (or soy sauce), ginger, rice vinegar, and 2 teaspoons water. Gently toss sauce with buckwheat (soba) noodles, salmon, shredded carrot, and spinach until coated.

Dinner

Grilled Chicken Tacos with Chipotle Cabbage Slaw

INGREDIENTS:

2 tsp mayonnaise

2 tsp lime juice

¼ tsp chipotle pepper powder

1 cup shredded red cabbage

1, 4-ounce cooked shredded chicken breast

2, 6-inch corn tortillas

⅛ of an avocado, cubed

fresh cilantro

PREPARATION: Whisk together mayonnaise, lime juice, chipotle pepper powder, and sea salt and toss with shredded purple cabbage. In a skillet with 1 teaspoon olive oil, over medium heat, heat corn tortillas until warmed, about one minute. Top each with half the chicken, ¼ of the slaw, ½ the avocado, and fresh cilantro (if you like it!). Serve with the remaining slaw on the side.

The Digestive Rest Diet

This plan is optimized to give your digestive system a rest by eliminating raw vegetables and dairy, which can be key culprits of digestive inflammation. It includes only a moderate amount of fruit each day. While the meals include vegetables, you'll notice that they also include a variety of other foods that provide important nutrients like protein, fat, and carbohydrates. This balance is not only important nutritionally, but it can also help to reduce stress on your digestive system. Your intake will be balanced in protein, minimally processed carbohydrates, and healthy fats to keep energy levels steady and strong. Lots of veggie lovers suffer from a case of "Too Much Raw Food," but fear not: this plan does not take away vegetables; it only takes away RAW vegetables. You will still be able to enjoy healthy, cooked favorites throughout the week.

DIGESTIVE REST SHOPPING LIST

Here is your grocery list! As promised, there is a lot of produce that you can buy. You'll be fully cooking all of these colorful vegetables in order to eliminate the inflammation that raw roughage causes in your system. Our recipes that follow will guide you through the preparation of these ingredients.

PRODUCE

Red onion (1 large)
Yellow onion (1 medium)

Grape tomatoes (2 cups)

Kale (1 bunch)

Sweet potato (3 medium)

Carrots (3 large)

Cremini mushrooms (1 cup, sliced)

Broccoli (2 heads)

Cauliflower (1 large head)

Green beans (2 cups)

Spaghetti squash (1 small squash, about 1 pound)

Garlic (3 cloves)

Avocado (1¼)

Basil (1 tablespoon, chopped)

Zucchini (1 small)

Pears (3 medium)

Orange (1)

Strawberries (¾ cup, sliced)

Bananas (3 large)

Blueberries (1 cup)

Grapes (at least 1 cup)

Lemon (1 small)

REFRIGERATED/DAIRY/MEAT

Eggs (6)

Bone-in, skin-on chicken thighs (2, 6-ounce each)

Wild salmon fillets (2, 6-ounce each)

Ground grass-fed beef or bison (8 ounces)

Peeled and cleaned shrimp (6 ounces)

Unsweetened almond milk (4 cups)

Salsa (¼ cup)

NON-PERISHABLES

Unsalted chicken or beef bone broth (5 cups)
Almond butter (½ cup)
Dark chocolate (chips or bar) (2½ ounces)
Full-fat canned coconut milk (1 cup)
Canned garbanzo beans (1½ cups)
Canned white beans (½ cup)
Unsweetened shredded coconut (2 teaspoons)
Sea salt potato chips (2 ounces)
Chopped walnuts (½ cup)
Chia seeds (¼ cup)
(Dark) chocolate-covered almonds (22)
Pumpkin seeds (¼ cup)
No-sugar-added marinara sauce (2 cups)
Salted cashews (2 tablespoons)
Raisins (2 tablespoons)
Tuna (1, 5-ounce can)
Sprouted grain bread (4 slices)
Quinoa (1⅓ cups)
Brown rice (1¼ cups)
Rolled oats (⅓ cup)

PANTRY ITEMS (YOU MAY ALREADY HAVE SOME OF THESE)

Olive oil (¾ cup)
Coconut oil (4 teaspoons)
Apple cider vinegar
Balsamic vinegar
Mustard

Garlic powder
Dried oregano
Curry powder
Ground turmeric
Sea salt
Black pepper
Ground ginger
Paprika
Ground cinnamon
Vanilla extract
Cocoa powder

RECIPES FOR SEVEN DAYS OF DIGESTIVE REST MEALS AND SNACKS

If you got mostly C's on the Diagnostic Nutrition Test, then the Digestive Rest Meal Plan is your best option.

DAY 1

Breakfast

Egg and Kale Scramble

INGREDIENTS:

2 eggs

3 tsp olive oil

¼ cup red onion, sliced

1½ cups chopped kale

1 slice of sprouted whole grain toast

PREPARATION: Whisk together the eggs and set aside. Heat 2 teaspoons of the olive oil in a medium skillet over medium heat, add the onion, and sauté until soft, about five minutes. Add the kale, and sauté until wilted, about three more minutes. Add eggs and cook, stirring occasionally, until firm, about three minutes. Serve with a slice of sprouted whole grain toast sprayed with the remaining teaspoon olive oil.

Lunch

Veggie Packed Bone Broth

INGREDIENTS:

3 cups unsalted chicken or beef bone broth

1 medium sweet potato, diced

(recipe continues)

½ cup carrot, diced

¼ tsp garlic powder

¼ tsp oregano

¼ tsp sea salt

⅓ cup chopped cremini mushrooms

½ cup broccoli florets

PREPARATION: In a saucepan, combine the chicken or beef broth with the sweet potato, garlic powder, oregano, and sea salt in a saucepan, and bring to a boil. Turn down to a simmer, cover, and cook until sweet potato is soft, about twenty minutes. Add the mushrooms and broccoli, cover, and simmer until broccoli is tender, about ten more minutes.

Dinner

Balsamic & Herb Roasted Chicken with Quinoa and Cauliflower

INGREDIENTS:

1½ tbsp balsamic vinegar

6 tsp olive oil

1 tsp dried oregano

½ tsp sea salt

¼ tsp black pepper

½ tsp garlic powder

2, 6-ounce bone-in, skin-on chicken thighs

4 cups of chopped cauliflower (florets and stems)

pinch of sea salt

pinch of black pepper

1¼ cups + 2 tablespoons quinoa

2⅔ cups water

PREPARATION: Preheat oven to 425 degrees F. Whisk together the balsamic vinegar, olive oil, oregano, sea salt, black pepper, and garlic powder. Pour mixture over the chicken thighs, and turn to coat. Line a baking dish with parchment paper, and place chicken thighs inside. Bake until chicken reaches an internal temperature of 165 degrees F, about twenty-five minutes.

Toss the cauliflower (florets and stems) with the olive oil and a pinch of sea salt and black pepper. Spread cauliflower out evenly on a baking sheet rubbed lightly with olive oil. Bake the cauliflower, stirring every ten minutes, until it's golden and soft, about twenty minutes.

While the chicken and cauliflower bake, bring the quinoa and water to a boil in a small sauce pan. Turn down to a simmer, cover, and cook until all water is absorbed, about twenty minutes. Serve one cup of the cooked quinoa topped with a chicken thigh and half the cauliflower. Store the remaining chicken thigh, half the cauliflower, and ½ cup quinoa for tomorrow's lunch. Refrigerate ¾ cup of the remaining quinoa for breakfast on Day 2, and freeze another ¾ cup for dinner on Day 5.

Snack

Pear with Almond Butter

Slice a pear in half and remove the seeds and stem. Spread 1½ teaspoons of almond butter onto each half.

Treat

Dark Chocolate-Coconut Vegan Truffle

Chop up 2½ ounces of dark chocolate (or use chocolate chips), and combine with 2 tablespoons full-fat canned coconut milk. Microwave for ten seconds, stir, and then microwave in five-second increments until the chocolate begins to soften, about fifteen more seconds, depending on your microwave. Stir until smooth and refrigerate until firm, about forty-five minutes. Scoop mixture out with a spoon and roll into three equal balls. Roll each in enough cocoa powder to coat (about 1 tablespoon cocoa powder total). Eat one truffle now, and refrigerate the other two for Days 4 and 7.

DAY 2

Breakfast

Strawberry-Walnut Quinoa Cereal

INGREDIENTS:
¾ cup leftover quinoa
¼ cup canned coconut milk
¼ cup unsweetened almond milk
½ cup sliced strawberries
1 tbsp chopped walnuts

PREPARATION: Combine ¾ cup of the leftover quinoa from dinner on Day 1 with the coconut milk and almond milk, and microwave just until heated, about thirty seconds. Top with the strawberries and walnuts.

Lunch

Leftover Balsamic Chicken, Cauliflower, and Quinoa

Re-heat last night's leftovers.

Dinner

Broccoli-Garbanzo Curry Bowl

INGREDIENTS:

1¼ cups brown rice

2½ cups water

1 cup sliced red onion

1 tbsp olive oil

2 tsp curry powder

¼ tsp sea salt

2 cups unsalted bone broth

4 cups roughly chopped broccoli

¼ cup canned coconut milk

1½ cups canned garbanzo beans

PREPARATION: Combine the brown rice and water in a sauce-pan, and bring to a boil. Turn down to a simmer, cover, and cook until all water is absorbed, about thirty minutes. While the rice cooks, sauté the onion in olive oil in a large skillet over medium-high heat, for about seven minutes. Once the onions are soft, add the curry powder, sea salt, and bone broth. Stir in the broccoli, and allow to simmer until broccoli begins

(recipe continues)

to soften, about ten minutes. Add the coconut milk and garbanzo beans. Simmer until the liquid has decreased by one-third and the broccoli begins to break apart, about ten more minutes. Serve half of the broccoli mixture over one cup of the cooked rice. Place the other half of the broccoli mixture over one cup of rice in a container to refrigerate for lunch on Day 3.

Snack

Banana with Almond Butter and Coconut

Cut ½ large banana into four equal pieces. Top one side of each piece with ½ teaspoon almond butter and ½ teaspoon shredded coconut.

Treat

Potato Chips

Enjoy 1 ounce (about 13 chips) organic sea salt potato chips (only ingredients should be potatoes, sea salt, and oil).

DAY 3

Breakfast

Blue Magic Smoothie

INGREDIENTS:
1 cup blueberries
½ ripe banana

¼ cup canned coconut milk

¼ tsp turmeric powder

¾ cup unsweetened almond milk

1 tbsp almond butter in a blender

PREPARATION: In a blender, combine the blueberries, banana, coconut milk, turmeric powder, almond milk, and almond butter. Blend until smooth. Add a handful of ice, and blend again until frothy.

Lunch

Broccoli-Garbanzo Curry Bowl (leftovers)

Have the leftover Broccoli-Garbanzo Curry Bowl from dinner on Day 2.

Dinner

Walnut-Crusted Salmon and Green Beans

INGREDIENTS:

¼ cup walnuts, chopped

¼ tsp dried oregano

⅛ tsp sea salt

1 tsp mustard

2, 6-ounce wild salmon fillets

2 cups green beans

1 tsp fresh lemon juice

¼ tsp lemon zest

1½ tsp olive oil

(recipe continues)

PREPARATION: Preheat the oven to 425 degrees F. Combine the walnuts with the oregano and sea salt. Spread the mustard onto each of the salmon fillets, and press half of the walnut mixture onto the top of each. Place the salmon fillets onto a parchment-paper-lined baking sheet, and bake at 425 until the fish flakes are done, about twenty minutes, checking at fifteen minutes.

While the fish cooks, steam the green beans until tender. Toss with the lemon juice and zest and the olive oil. Serve one salmon fillet with one cup of the green beans. Refrigerate the other salmon fillet and one cup of the green beans for lunch on Day 4.

Prep Ahead

Roasted Sweet Potatoes

Dice 2 medium sweet potatoes (about 3 cups total), toss with 4 teaspoons coconut oil and a ½ teaspoon sea salt, and place on a baking sheet in the oven until potato is soft and golden, about thirty minutes, stirring every fifteen minutes. Refrigerate the roasted sweet potato for lunch on Day 4, dinner on Day 6, and lunch on Day 7.

Prep Ahead

Chia Pudding

Combine ¼ cup chia seeds with 1½ cups unsweetened almond milk and ½ teaspoon vanilla extract. Cover and refrigerate until breakfast tomorrow.

Hard-Boiled Egg with Pumpkin Seeds

Eat one hard-boiled egg with 2 tablespoons pumpkin seeds.

Treat

(Dark) Chocolate-Covered Almonds

Eat 11 chocolate-covered almonds.

DAY 4

Breakfast

Strawberry-Banana and Almond Butter Chia Pudding

Pour half of the chia pudding mixture you made last night into a bowl. Stir in one mashed banana and 1 tablespoon almond butter. Top with ¼ cup sliced strawberries.

Lunch

Roasted Sweet Potato with Green Beans and Walnut Salmon

Toss the leftover green beans with 1 cup roasted sweet potato, the leftover walnut salmon, and 1 tablespoon pumpkin seeds.

Dinner

Spaghetti Squash with Beef Marinara Sauce

INGREDIENTS:

1 small spaghetti squash (about 1 pound)

½ cup yellow onion, chopped

1 tbsp olive oil

¼ tsp sea salt

1 clove of garlic, crushed or diced

¼ tsp dried oregano

⅛ tsp black pepper

8 ounces ground grass-fed beef (or ground bison)

2 cups no-sugar-added marinara sauce

PREPARATION: Preheat oven to 400 degrees F. Cut the spaghetti squash in half from end to end. Scoop out the seeds with a spoon and place the squash, cut side down, in a baking dish with at least one-inch sides large enough to fit both squash halves. Pour enough water to fill one-eighth-inch deep in the baking dish. Bake until the squash is tender, about forty minutes.

While the squash cooks, sauté the onion in the olive oil until tender, about five minutes. Add the sea salt, garlic, oregano, black pepper, and the beef. Cook until the ground beef is lightly browned, stirring to break up any chunks, about five minutes. Add the marinara sauce, and continue to simmer until the mixture thickens, about five more minutes.

Using a fork, scrape the squash flesh from the skin to form long strings. Place half of the squash onto a plate and top with half of the ground beef sauce. Place the other half of the

squash and sauce in a container, and refrigerate for lunch on
Day 5.

> **NOTE:** *Remove quinoa from the freezer to use for dinner on*
> *Day 5.*

Snack

Cashews and Raisins

Combine 2 tablespoons lightly salted cashews and 2 tablespoons seedless raisins.

Treat

Hot Chocolate

Heat up ½ cup of unsweetened almond milk until steaming
hot. Pour into a mug with one of the chocolate truffles made
on Day 1. Stir to dissolve.

DAY 5

Breakfast

Avocado Toast with Hard-Boiled Egg

INGREDIENTS:
1 slice of sprouted grain bread
¼ avocado
1 hard-boiled egg

(recipe continues)

salt and pepper, as desired

1 small orange, sliced

PREPARATION: Toast the bread, spread with the avocado, and then top with the egg. Season with salt and pepper as desired. Serve with a small orange, sliced.

Lunch

Spaghetti Squash with Beef Marinara (leftovers)

Eat the leftover spaghetti squash with beef marinara from dinner on Day 4.

Dinner

Garlic-Basil Shrimp with Grape Tomatoes and Carrot Fries

INGREDIENTS:

2 large carrots

1 tbsp + 2 tsp olive oil

pinch of sea salt

pinch of black pepper

6 ounces shrimp, peeled and cleaned

1 clove garlic, crushed and chopped

1 tbsp sliced fresh basil

2 tbsp balsamic vinegar

leftover, thawed quinoa

PREPARATION: Preheat oven to 425 degrees F. Slice the carrots into three to four long sticks. Toss with the olive oil and a pinch of sea salt and black pepper. Place in a single layer on a baking sheet, and bake until tender and golden, fifteen to twenty minutes.

Heat the olive oil over medium-high heat. Add the shrimp, and cook until they just start to turn opaque, three to four minutes, flipping shrimp halfway through to brown evenly on both sides. Add the grape tomatces, garlic, basil, and balsamic vinegar, stirring ingredients to release any browned bits from the bottom.

Cook until shrimp is firm and completely opaque, about another minute. Remove shrimp from the pan and add the thawed quinoa. Cook on low heat until warmed through. Serve shrimp over quinoa with half the carrot fries on the side.

Refrigerate half the carrot fries for lunch on Day 6.

Prep Ahead

Overnight Oats

Prepare overnight oats for breakfast on Day 6: combine half a banana, mashed, with 2 teaspoons almond butter, a pinch of ground ginger, ¾ cup unsweetened almond milk, and ¾ cup rolled oats in a jar, and stir to combine. Refrigerate overnight.

Snack

Pear Chia Pudding

Pour half the remaining chia pudding into a bowl and top with ½ a chopped pear.

Treat

(Dark) Chocolate-Covered Almonds

11 chocolate-covered almonds OR pair 11 almonds with ½-ounce dark chocolate.

DAY 6

Breakfast

Pear-Pumpkin-Seed Overnight Oats

Top the overnight oats made last night with half a pear, diced, and 1 tablespoon pumpkin seeds.

Lunch

Avocado Tuna Salad Sandwich with Carrot Fries

INGREDIENTS:
1, 3-ounce drained canned tuna
½ avocado, lightly mashed
1 tsp lemon juice

2 tsp pumpkin seeds
salt and black pepper to taste
2 slices of sprouted grain bread
leftover carrot fries

PREPARATION: Combine the tuna with the avocado, lemon juice, pumpkin seeds, and salt and black pepper to taste. Sandwich tuna salad between two slices of sprouted grain bread, and serve with leftover carrot fries from dinner on Day 5.

Dinner

Kale and Mushroom Omelet

INGREDIENTS:
3 tsp olive oil
¼ cup yellow onion, chopped
½ cup sliced cremini mushrooms
1 cup of chopped kale
⅛ tsp sea salt
2 eggs
1 tbsp unsweetened almond milk

PREPARATION: Heat 2 teaspoons of the olive oil in a medium skillet over medium heat. Add the onion and mushrooms, and cook until soft, about six minutes. Add the kale and sea salt. Cook until kale is wilted, about two more minutes. Remove from pan and set aside.

Whisk the eggs and almond milk in a bowl. Add another teaspoon olive oil to the pan in which you cooked the veggies,

(recipe continues)

and heat over medium heat. Add the egg mixture to the pan, and allow to cook until firm, gently scraping in from the edges for even cooking. Add the veggie mixture to one half, and fold the egg round in half to form an omelet. In the same skillet, heat half the leftover sweet potato until warmed through, and serve next to the omelet.

NOTE: *Thaw the chicken from Day 1 to use for dinner tomorrow.*

Prep Ahead

Steamed Broccoli

Steam one cup broccoli for lunch on Day 7.

Snack

Almond Butter and Pumpkin-Seed Banana Slices

Slice half a banana into four rounds. Top each round with ½ teaspoon almond butter, and then press each into 1 teaspoon pumpkin seeds.

Treat

Potato Chips

Enjoy 1 ounce (about 13 chips) organic sea salt potato chips (only ingredients should be potatoes, sea salt, and oil).

DAY 7

Breakfast

Avocado Baked Egg with Salsa

INGREDIENTS:
½ avocado
¼ cup salsa
1 egg
pinch of sea salt
pinch of black pepper
½ pear
1 tbsp almond butter

PREPARATION: Preheat oven to 350 degrees F. Slice an avocado in half, and scoop out enough of the flesh in one half, around where the pit was, to allow an egg white and yolk to fit. Combine any avocado flesh you scooped out with the salsa and set aside. Crack an egg into the center of the avocado half, and sprinkle with a pinch of sea salt and black pepper. Bake at 350 until the egg is firm, about fifteen minutes. Serve topped with the salsa-avocado mixture and half a pear spread with the almond butter on the side.

Lunch

Sweet Potato and White Bean Salad

INGREDIENTS:

2 tsp olive oil

2 tsp lemon juice

¼ tsp lemon zest

⅛ tsp sea salt

pinch of black pepper

pinch of paprika

½ cup canned white beans, rinsed and drained

1 cup steamed broccoli

1 cup leftover roasted sweet potatoes

1 tbsp walnuts, chopped

PREPARATION: Whisk together the olive oil, lemon juice and zest, sea salt, and a pinch each of black pepper and paprika. Set aside. Toss together the white beans, broccoli, the final cup of leftover roasted sweet potatoes, the walnuts, and the lemon and oil dressing. Toss to coat.

Dinner

Zoodles with Garlic-Almond Butter Sauce

INGREDIENTS:

1 small-medium zucchini, or about 1 cup of zucchini "noodles"

1 tbsp olive oil

1 cup of grape tomatoes

⅛ tsp salt

pinch of black pepper
leftover chicken thigh
1½ tbsp almond butter
2 tsp apple cider vinegar
1 tsp water
1 clove of garlic, crushed and diced
⅛ tsp sea salt

PREPARATION: Use a julienne peeler or a spiralizer to create the zucchini strands, or "noodles." In a medium skillet, heat the olive oil over medium-high heat. Add the zucchini noodles and cook, stirring often, until they begin to soften, about eight minutes. Add the grape tomatoes, salt, and a pinch of black pepper. Add the leftover chicken thigh, and continue to cook until tomatoes crack open, about five more minutes. Cook over low heat until the chicken is warmed through, and stir in the cooked spaghetti. Stir together the almond butter, apple cider vinegar, water, garlic, and sea salt. Pour the almond butter mixture over the zucchini mixture and toss to coat.

Snack

Pear-Cinnamon Chia Pudding

Stir ⅛ teaspoon ground cinnamon into the remaining ½ cup chia pudding, and top with ½ chopped pear.

Treat

Dark Chocolate-Coconut Truffle

Eat the last truffle!

DIGESTIVE REST BONUS DAYS

DAY 1

Breakfast

Open-Faced Egg and Greens Sandwich

INGREDIENTS:
1 slice of whole grain sprouted toast
1 tbsp hummus
1½ tsp olive oil
1 egg
1½ cups baby spinach
1 small orange

PREPARATION: Heat a medium skillet over medium heat. Add olive oil and cook egg until desired doneness is reached, about two minutes on each side for over medium. Remove egg from pan and set aside. Add ½ teaspoon olive oil to the skillet. Sauté the spinach until wilted, about one minute.

Spread the hummus over the toast. Top with egg and spinach. Serve with 1 small orange.

Lunch

Mediterranean Quinoa Salad Bowl with Chicken

INGREDIENTS:

½ cup cooked quinoa

¼ cup rinsed and drained canned chickpeas

1, 3-ounce boneless grilled chicken

½ cup chopped roasted peppers

2 tbsp chopped parsley

2 tbsp olive oil

1 tsp lemon juice

1 tsp white wine vinegar

⅛ tsp salt

⅛ tsp cumin

dash of cayenne pepper

PREPARATION: Toss quinoa with chickpeas, roasted peppers, and chopped parsley. Dress with olive oil whisked lemon juice, white wine vinegar, salt, cumin, and dash of cayenne pepper.

Dinner

Grass-Fed Beef Burger with Roasted Zucchini and Onions

INGREDIENTS:

½ zucchini cut into ¼ inch thick rounds

½ medium onion, sliced

¼ tsp salt, divided

(recipe continues)

1 tsp balsamic vinegar

pinch ground black pepper

1, 4-ounce grass-fed ground beef

3 tsp olive oil, divided

1 whole grain hamburger bun

1 tbsp hummus

PREPARATION: Preheat oven to 400 degrees F. Spread the onions and zucchini evenly on a baking sheet and toss with two teaspoons olive oil. Bake for ten minutes then flip zucchini over. Bake another five minutes or until veggies are tender. Add balsamic vinegar, salt, and black pepper to a mixing bowl. Stir in beef and mix until spices are evenly distributed. Form into a patty about ¼ inch thick.

Heat a skillet over medium-high heat. Add one teaspoon olive oil and place patty into the pan. Cook until desired doneness, flipping once. About three minutes on each side will yield medium.

Place the burger on the bun, spread with hummus and top with roasted zucchini and onion. Serve any remaining vegetables on the side.

DAY 2

Breakfast

Raspberry Almond Butter Sweet Potato Toast

INGREDIENTS:

4, ⅛ inch thick slices sweet potato

2 tbsp almond butter

½ cup halved raspberries
cinnamon (optional)

PREPARATION: Place the sweet potato slices in the toaster and toast until soft and golden, about four toasting cycles. Spread each slice with ½ tablespoon almond butter and two tablespoons raspberries. Add cinnamon if desired.

Lunch

Egg Salad with Grapes and Walnuts

INGREDIENTS:
2 hard boiled eggs
1 tbsp regular mayonnaise
1 tsp lemon juice
1 cup grapes, divided
2 tbsp finely chopped walnuts
black pepper to taste
sea salt to taste
¼ avocado, sliced
2 slices whole wheat bread
1 cup grapes, divided

PREPARATION: Lightly mash hard boiled eggs and stir in mayonnaise and lemon juice. Stir in ¼ cup of the grapes cut into halves or quarters, and the walnuts. Add black pepper and salt to taste. Place egg salad on one slice of bread, then top with sliced avocado. Serve with remaining grapes on the side.

Dinner

Grilled Lamb Chops, Sweet Potato Fries, and Broccoli

INGREDIENTS:

1, 4-ounce lamb chop

½ medium sweet potato

3 tsp olive oil, divided

¼ tsp salt

¼ tsp cumin

⅛ tsp cinnamon

⅛ tsp black pepper

2 cups broccoli florets

1 tsp lemon juice

¼ tsp lemon zest

    (optional but recommended for lots of flavor)

PREPARATION: Pre-heat oven to 400 degrees F. Chop the sweet potato into fry-shaped pieces. Toss sweet potatoes with two teaspoons olive oil and arrange evenly on a baking sheet. Bake until crisp, about twenty minutes, turning halfway through cooking time.

While sweet potatoes cook, pat lamb dry with paper towels (this helps produce a nice golden crust as it cooks). Rub both sides with the blend of salt, pepper, cumin, and cinnamon. Heat a grill or grill pan over medium high heat. Grill lamb chops about four to five minutes per side or until cooked to 145 degrees F for medium rare.

Steam broccoli florets and toss with one teaspoon lemon juice, ¼ teaspoon lemon zest, and one teaspoon olive oil. Serve lamb chops with fries and broccoli.

DAY 3

Breakfast

Strawberry-Walnut Chia Pudding

INGREDIENTS:

3 tbsp chia seeds

1 cup unsweetened vanilla almond milk

¼ ripe banana, mashed

⅛ tsp cinnamon

¾ cup sliced or chopped strawberries

1 tbsp chopped walnuts

PREPARATION: Whisk chia seeds with almond milk, banana, and cinnamon. Let the mixture sit, covered, in the fridge for at least two hours or overnight.

Top with chopped walnuts, strawberries, and a sprinkle of cinnamon, if desired.

Lunch

Lentil Grain Bowl

INGREDIENTS:

½ cup cooked green or brown lentils

1½ cups cauliflower

¾ cup cooked farro or other whole grain

¼ of an avocado, chopped

1 tsp olive oil

1 tsp balsamic vinegar

(recipe continues)

PREPARATION: Preheat oven to 400 degrees F. Toss cauliflower in two teaspoons olive oil, then spread evenly on a baking sheet. Cook for ten minutes, then turn over and cook for another five minutes, or until cauliflower is golden and tender.

Place lentils and farro in a bowl and top with cauliflower, avocado, and oil and vinegar.

Dinner

Chicken and Vegetable Cacciatore

INGREDIENTS:

1, 4-ounce chicken breast, cut into ½-inch cubes
1 tsp olive oil
⅓ cup chopped onion
⅓ cup chopped red bell pepper
⅓ cup sliced mushroom
½ tsp chopped garlic
2 tbsp dry white wine
1 cup canned diced tomatoes
⅛ tsp dried oregano
⅛ tsp salt
1 cup cooked whole wheat pasta

PREPARATION: Sauté chicken breast in one teaspoon olive oil until browned on outside. Remove chicken from pan and set aside. Add onion, red pepper, and sliced mushroom and cook until vegetables soften, about five minutes. Add garlic, white wine, and diced tomatoes (not drained), oregano, salt, and a dash of red pepper flakes (optional). Simmer for about ten minutes; add chicken and simmer another five minutes (until chicken is fully cooked). Serve over whole wheat pasta. Top with one teaspoon grated Parmesan cheese.

PART III

MAINTAINING YOUR BACK-DIET CONNECTION

6.

LONG-TERM ADVICE: HOW TO CONTINUE FEELING GREAT

1. *Keep symptom journals.*

   It's important to keep track of how you're feeling throughout the entire process of following a meal plan. We recommend rating your back pain and digestive symptoms on a scale of 0 to 10 (0=non-existent pain, 10=extremely severe pain) and keeping notes each day. Your symptom notes can be written directly into your food journal. The goal of each diet plan is to achieve daily symptom scores of 2 or lower.

2. *Wait until all symptoms are at a score of 2 or lower for a full month before you start reintroducing new foods.*

   If you start to reintroduce foods before you've had a full month with limited symptoms, it will be difficult to tell exactly what food or drink is your trigger for symptoms.

3. *Introduce only one new food at a time and give your-self two weeks to track potential reactions.*

   A reaction to a food or drink can happen a couple hours after eating/drinking or a couple of days later. For this reason, it's important to introduce just one new food at a time and to give yourself at least two weeks with that food being added back into your diet in order to see if your symptom ratings on your food records have changed.

4. *Don't rush the process.*

   After you introduce a new food or drink, even if you don't have a reaction, remove it while you introduce the next one. This prevents a cumulative effect of foods that may not cause a reaction by themselves but do when eaten close together.

5. *Test combinations of foods last.*

   Once you've reintroduced all foods one by one and made a list of those foods that are triggers for adverse symptoms and those foods that are not triggers, it's time to test combinations of those two food groups.

   Test one combination at a time, and give yourself two full days before trying out the next combination. Once you know which foods can be combined and still sit well with you, you can try eating three of the rein-troduced foods all at once. However, we still encour-age you to follow the guidelines for things like alcohol, sugar, and caffeine outlined below. A basic combining test may look like this:

Day One: reintroduced food A + reintroduced food B

Day Four: reintroduced food C + reintroduced food D

Day Seven: A + B + C

Day Ten: A + B + D

Etc.

6. *If you already know a specific food is a trigger food for symptoms, do not include that in your reintroduction.*

    If you have been lactose intolerant for years, do not attempt to add dairy back into your diet. If you've been diagnosed with celiac disease or non-celiac gluten intolerance, do not introduce gluten. If you've always felt very shaky or gotten heartburn after drinking coffee, don't add it back in. These, unfortunately, are no-no's for you, medically speaking, and these are the few foods that you will have to live without!

7. *Don't eat it just because it's "good" for you.*

    Not a big drinker but heard about all the heart health benefits of alcohol? Health-wise, it's not worth starting to drink. Not a fan of the flavor of kale but know all the healthy folks on Instagram are obsessed with it? Opt for spinach or arugula or another green leafy veggie you do love. A large part of feeling good and developing a healthy relationship with food is enjoying what you eat.

WILL ALCOHOL, CAFFEINE, SUGAR, AND REFINED CARBS BE ALLOWED BACK INTO MY DIET?

Yes, as long as these are not major triggers for your symptoms. If you find they do not trigger painful or unpleasant symptoms, here are the guidelines for how much of these foods you can include in your diet in a healthful, balanced way:

Alcohol: Limiting alcohol each day is important for your heart health as well as the healthy functioning of all of your organs and systems. Limit alcohol to no more than one drink per day for women and no more than two drinks per day for men. A drink is one 12-ounce beer, 4 ounces of wine, 1.5 ounces of 80-proof spirits, or 1 ounce of 100-proof spirits. Also, alcohol and refined carbs fall into the same category, so if you are sensitive to either of these things, you can alternate to keep your body from getting too much. For example, enjoy refined carbs one day, but skip the booze that day, and vice versa.

Refined carbs: Refined carbs are those that have been processed in a way that removes the fiber and, therefore, most of the nutrition. An example would be white flour made from wheat. The wheat germ (which houses the fiber and B vitamins) has been removed, and you're left mainly with carbohydrate and little else. Products made with refined grains should be limited to one hundred calories each day. This could be a small white flour roll at dinner, a few crackers or pretzels at a work meeting, or a small portion of a dessert made with white flour.

Coffee/caffeine: Keep caffeine intake under 400 mg each day. The cutoff for caffeine is two p.m., because caffeine sticks around in your system for about eight hours after you ingest it. We don't want that afternoon cup of joe (or even tea) messing with your sleep! The limit for coffee is two 10-ounce cups of homemade coffee each day (or one grande Starbucks coffee or two grande espresso drinks, such as lattes). Tea varies in its caffeine content, but in general, green and black teas have about 50 mg of caffeine per 8-ounce cup.

Sugar: Sugar intake includes ALL sweeteners, such as honey, maple syrup, white sugar, coconut sugar, molasses, etc. Daily added sugar intake should stay below six teaspoons for women and no more than nine teaspoons for men. For easy reference, there are four grams of sugar per teaspoon. That means that if you are eating a chocolate bar, sweetened with coconut sugar, and it has twelve grams of sugar, you are eating three teaspoons of your daily sugar allotment (twelve grams divided by four grams/teaspoons = three teaspoons of sugar).

WHAT ABOUT THE HEALTHIER FOODS THAT THE DIETS CUT OUT?

All three diets cut out processed sugar, processed carbs, and alcohol (see recommendations above). However, in addition to these less nutrient-rich foods, each diet cut out some more nutritious options as well. Here is a reminder of what specifically was cut from each plan.

THE PALEO PLUS DIET

Cut: Alcohol, caffeine, processed sugar, gluten, dairy
Limited: Grains and beans

THE FODMAPS DIET

Cut: Dairy, gluten, pears, apples, cherries, raspberries, blackberries, watermelon, nectarines, peaches, apricots, plums, prunes, mango, papaya, persimmon, orange juice, canned fruit, artichokes, asparagus, sugar snap peas, cabbage, onion, shallot, leek, onions, garlic, cauliflower, mushrooms, pumpkin, green peppers, wheat, rye, barley, spelt, beans and lentils, pistachios, honey, agave, high fructose corn syrup, sorbitol, mannitol, xylitol, maltitol, Splenda, inulin, FOS, sugar alcohols, chicory root

Limited: Fruit (no more than one serving per meal); dried fruit (no more than one tablespoon per day); avocado (no more than one-quarter avocado per day); less than one-half cup sweet potato, broccoli, Brussels sprouts, butternut squash, or fennel each day; less than ten snow peas per day; no more than ten nuts (almonds, macadamia, pecans, pine nuts, walnuts, pumpkin seeds, sesame seeds, sunflower seeds) per day; and no more than one cup of coffee per day

THE DIGESTIVE REST DIET

Cut: Raw vegetables, refined grains, dairy, coffee
Limited: No more than two cups of fruit per day

Here's how to add back the more nutritious options:

1. Add the foods that were cut, one at a time, according to the instructions and guidelines above.

2. Increase the portions and/or number of times you eat each of the foods that were limited daily over the course of the two-week testing period, and monitor your symptoms as you eat more. Adding back a small amount of a food that had been limited might not give you any symptoms, but a lot might, and that will be your way to establish how much of a certain food you can eat and still maintain your health. FODMAPS sufferers tend to have the most immediate reactions, so here are my portion recommendations for reintroduction:

   - Fructose—½ mango or 1 to 2 teaspoons honey
   - Fructans—2 slices wheat bread, 1 garlic clove, or 1 cup pasta
   - Galactans—½ cup lentils or chickpeas
   - Sugar Alcohols—Sorbitol, 2 to 4 dried apricots; mannitol, ½ cup mushrooms
   - Lactose—Dairy requires a more scientific reintroduction. The lactose (the sugar in dairy foods that can cause digestive symptoms in some people) levels vary within the dairy foods category. Aged cheeses—like cheddar, Parmesan, and Swiss—tend to have less lactose than fresh cheeses like feta and ricotta. And yogurt has less lactose than fluid milk. When reintroducing dairy, we recommend starting with the lower lactose dairy first, such as aged cheeses and yogurt, before trying fresh cheeses or fluid milk. When you do work your way up to milk, start with just one-half to one- cup.

REINTRODUCTION FAQs

Here are some quick answers to many of the Frequently Asked Questions that nutritionists Jarosh and Clarke receive in their practice:

Q: *What happens if I eat a bunch of my trigger foods in one day, or go way overboard with portions, and my symptoms come back?*

A: Because this does happen, the most important thing you can do is not beat yourself up. Halloween, Thanksgiving, and Christmas happen! Return to eating from the meal plans in this book for a week post-holiday or post-"cheat" to get your symptoms back to a score of 2 or lower on the scale of 1 to 10. Then, return to a balanced diet, with the foods you've already tested and know work for you, in the amounts you know make you feel good.

Q: *Can I still dine out and follow these eating plans?*

A: Yes! We recommend limiting dining out to no more than two times per week while following these plans. This ensures that you know exactly what is going into your meals and snacks. It will likely take a bit more planning on your part and maybe some flexibility with your fellow diners regarding where you eat, but it is completely doable. Look up the restaurant's menu online ahead of time, and make choices that follow the general guidelines in terms of foods that are not included in the diet and those that are allowed in limited quantities. As long as your meal fulfills those guidelines, you are still following the plan!

We also recommend calling the restaurant ahead of time if you have questions about ingredients, or any diet-related questions. And don't be shy when you're placing your order—ask for what you want! It's always better to ask, even if your server reports back that the kitchen cannot fulfill a certain special request. But be prepared, and have a backup choice as well.

Q: *What if I have to travel while I'm following these plans?*

A: Do as much research as you can about the restaurants available at your destination. Also, research grocery stores in the area, so you can pick up general supplies to keep in the mini-fridge of your hotel room. When planning airport travel, try to have breakfast at home (or pack it), and pack lunch and snacks. When eating on the road, be sure to refer to the foods that are not allowed on each plan, as well as those that are limited, and stick to those guidelines.

Q: *How much water should I drink while on these meal plans?*

A: There is no hard and fast rule that works for everyone, because we all have slightly different hydration needs, depending on height, weight, activity level, diet, and climate. Start with eight 8-ounce glasses of water each day (more during workouts), and increase as needed in order to keep your urine pale yellow/clear all day long. If your urine is darker, like the color of apple juice, it likely means you're dehydrated and need to drink more water.

Q: *Can I work out on these plans?*

A: Yes! These plans are rich in nutrients and have the correct balance of protein, carbohydrate, and healthy fats to fuel workouts. Individual needs may vary, so if you find that you're becoming too hungry throughout the day, then add an additional snack or double the size of your snack.

Q: *What if I'm too full or too hungry on these plans?*

A: If you find that you're becoming too full on these plans, try cutting your lunch and/or dinner in half. Save the other half to use as an additional snack in case you get hungrier. If you're getting too hungry, add an additional snack or double the size of your snack each day.

It's important to listen to your body's s natural fullness cues, and stop eating when you're satisfied (but before you become full). This is why, rather than cut out snacks, we prefer to reduce the size of meals if you're feeling too full on the plans. Snacks are a great way to add the daily nutrition that you may not get at meals and also allow you to eat just until you're satisfied at mealtime. You can feel confident that if you get hungry before your next meal, you can eat your snack.

7.

RECORDING YOUR SYMPTOMS

Nutritionists Willow Jarosh and Stephanie Clarke recommend that all their clients keep a Symptom Journal to help identify patterns in input, output, and pain and also to determine if particular symptoms are the result of a specific food—or possibly something else! In this section, you will find a handy Symptom Journal to help you record all of the information necessary to pinpoint the source of your digestive pain and track your progress as you follow one of the prescribed Back Pain Relief Diets. Feel free to make notes in your phone or another journal or diary if that feels more comfortable. The most important thing is recording the information—not where you keep it! If you decide to record your food journey elsewhere, please do have a look at the Symptom Journal notes and prompts that follow so that you are familiar with the types of things you should be writing down.

SYMPTOM JOURNAL NOTES

Here are a few explanatory notes to help you best fill out the Symptom Journal:

IDENTIFYING YOUR HUNGER

You will be asked to rank your hunger both before and after each meal. This is important because it might help you identify when you are eating as a result of stress or boredom or when you have gotten too hungry and have ended up eating more than your system can handle at one time. Ranking your hunger can also help you identify which foods make you feel really great and which ones make you feel too full and uncomfortable—even if you haven't had a large portion! Rank your hunger on a scale of 1 to 10: 1 = starving, 10 = stuffed.

GUIDANCE FOR YOUR "DIGESTIVE NOTES"

After each meal, you will be prompted to make digestive notes to provide more detail about how you feel after eating. This is one of the keys to identifying your allergens and inflammatory foods and also assessing how the hunger scale relates to your symptoms. Please listen to your body. Are you bloated? Do you feel gassy? Do you have to run to the restroom? Do you have stomach pains? Whatever you feel, write it down!

GUIDANCE FOR YOUR "END-OF-DAY BODY NOTES"

After each meal, you will be recording the specifics of what you ate, how much, and how you felt, but at the end of each day, it's also important to note what else your body endured that day and how it is feeling in general. You'll want to note the quality of your sleep from the night before, the amount and type of exercise you performed, your energy level, the number and type of bowel movements you had using the Stool Chart in Chapter 2, and overall pain notes. If your back is feeling better, note it! If it's feeling worse, note it! Ideally, with all of this additional information, we'll be able to find a pattern in your overall self-care and body response and help pinpoint specifically your sources of discomfort or pain!

NOTE YOUR MEALTIME!

We encourage you to write down what time you eat each meal. This may not seem important, but some people have a wildly erratic meal schedule due to late meetings, long hours, and the daily distractions and responsibilities of life. It can really benefit the body to create a meal and snack schedule to help your system regulate, keep your metabolism stable, and prevent your body from getting too hungry. Sometimes seeing *on paper* how long you actually go between meals and snacks can be a gentle reminder to grab your snack for that long meeting and keep your body—and your digestive system—functioning optimally!

Symptom Journal

■

DAY 1

Breakfast

Time of Meal _____

Hunger Prior to Eating _____

Food and Drink Consumed/Quantities _____

_____

_____

_____

_____

Hunger Post-Meal _____

Digestive Notes _____

_____

_____

_____

_____

Lunch

Time of Meal _____

Hunger Prior to Eating _____

Food and Drink Consumed/Quantities _____

_____

_____

_____

_____

Hunger Post-Meal _____

Digestive Notes _____

_____

_____

_____

_____

Dinner

Time of Meal _____

Hunger Prior to Eating _____

Food and Drink Consumed/Quantities _____

_____

_____

_____

_____

Hunger Post-Meal _____

Digestive Notes _____

_____

_____

_____

_____

End-Of-Day Body Notes

Hours of Sleep _____

Bowel Movements _____

_____

Exercise _____

_____

_____

_____

Overall Pain _____

_____

_____

_____

DAY 2

Breakfast

Time of Meal _____

Hunger Prior to Eating _____

Food and Drink Consumed/Quantities _____

_____

_____

_____

_____

Hunger Post-Meal _____

Digestive Notes _____

_____

_____

_____

_____

Lunch

Time of Meal _____

Hunger Prior to Eating _____

Food and Drink Consumed/Quantities _____

_____

_____

_____

Hunger Post-Meal _____

Digestive Notes _____

_____

_____

_____

_____

Dinner

Time of Meal _____

Hunger Prior to Eating _____

Food and Drink Consumed/Quantities _____

_____

_____

_____

_____

Hunger Post-Meal _____

Digestive Notes _____

_____

_____

_____

End-Of-Day Body Notes

Hours of Sleep _____

Bowel Movements _____

_____

Exercise _____

_____

_____

_____

Overall Pain _____

_____

_____

_____

JOURNAL

DAY 3

Breakfast

Time of Meal _____

Hunger Prior to Eating _____

Food and Drink Consumed/Quantities _____

_____

_____

_____

_____

Hunger Post-Meal _____

Digestive Notes _____

_____

_____

_____

_____

Lunch

Time of Meal _____

Hunger Prior to Eating _____

Food and Drink Consumed/Quantities _____

_____

_____

_____

Hunger Post-Meal _____

Digestive Notes _____

_____

_____

_____

_____

Dinner

Time of Meal _____

Hunger Prior to Eating _____

Food and Drink Consumed/Quantities _____

_____

_____

_____

_____

Hunger Post-Meal _____

Digestive Notes _____

_____

_____

_____

_____

End-Of-Day Body Notes

Hours of Sleep _____

Bowel Movements _____

_____

Exercise _____

_____

_____

_____

Overall Pain _____

_____

_____

_____

DAY 4

Breakfast

Time of Meal _____

Hunger Prior to Eating _____

Food and Drink Consumed/Quantities _____

_____

_____

_____

_____

Hunger Post-Meal _____

Digestive Notes _____

_____

_____

_____

_____

Lunch

Time of Meal _____

Hunger Prior to Eating _____

Food and Drink Consumed/Quantities _____

_____

_____

_____

Hunger Post-Meal _____

Digestive Notes _____

_____

_____

_____

_____

Dinner

Time of Meal _____

Hunger Prior to Eating _____

Food and Drink Consumed/Quantities _____

_____

_____

_____

_____

Hunger Post-Meal _____

Digestive Notes _____

_____

_____

_____

_____

End-Of-Day Body Notes

Hours of Sleep _____

Bowel Movements _____

_____

Exercise _____

_____

_____

_____

Overall Pain _____

_____

_____

_____

DAY 5

Breakfast

Time of Meal _____

Hunger Prior to Eating _____

Food and Drink Consumed/Quantities _____

_____

_____

_____

_____

Hunger Post-Meal _____

Digestive Notes _____

_____

_____

_____

_____

Lunch

Time of Meal _____

Hunger Prior to Eating _____

Food and Drink Consumed/Quantities _____

_____

_____

_____

Hunger Post-Meal _____

Digestive Notes _____

_____

_____

_____

_____

Dinner

Time of Meal _____

Hunger Prior to Eating _____

Food and Drink Consumed/Quantities _____

_____

_____

_____

_____

Hunger Post-Meal _____

Digestive Notes _____

_____

_____

_____

_____

End-Of-Day Body Notes

Hours of Sleep _____

Bowel Movements _____

_____

Exercise _____

_____

_____

_____

Overall Pain _____

_____

_____

_____

DAY 6

Breakfast

Time of Meal _____

Hunger Prior to Eating _____

Food and Drink Consumed/Quantities _____

_____

_____

_____

_____

Hunger Post-Meal _____

Digestive Notes _____

_____

_____

_____

_____

Lunch

Time of Meal _____

Hunger Prior to Eating _____

Food and Drink Consumed/Quantities _____

_____

_____

_____

Hunger Post-Meal _____

Digestive Notes _____

_____

_____

_____

_____

Dinner

Time of Meal _____

Hunger Prior to Eating _____

Food and Drink Consumed/Quantities _____

_____

_____

_____

_____

Hunger Post-Meal _____

Digestive Notes _____

_____

_____

_____

_____

End-Of-Day Body Notes

Hours of Sleep _____

Bowel Movements _____
_____

Exercise _____
_____
_____
_____

Overall Pain _____
_____
_____

DAY 7

Breakfast

Time of Meal _____

Hunger Prior to Eating _____

Food and Drink Consumed/Quantities _____

_____

_____

_____

_____

Hunger Post-Meal _____

Digestive Notes _____

_____

_____

_____

_____

Lunch

Time of Meal _____

Hunger Prior to Eating _____

Food and Drink Consumed/Quantities _____

_____

_____

_____

Hunger Post-Meal _____

Digestive Notes _____

_____

_____

_____

_____

Dinner

Time of Meal _____

Hunger Prior to Eating _____

Food and Drink Consumed/Quantities _____

_____

_____

_____

_____

Hunger Post-Meal _____

Digestive Notes _____

_____

_____

_____

_____

End-Of-Day Body Notes

Hours of Sleep _____

Bowel Movements _____

_____

Exercise _____

_____

_____

_____

Overall Pain _____

_____

_____

_____

DAY 8

Breakfast

Time of Meal _____

Hunger Prior to Eating _____

Food and Drink Consumed/Quantities _____

_____

_____

_____

_____

Hunger Post-Meal _____

Digestive Notes _____

_____

_____

_____

_____

Lunch

Time of Meal _____

Hunger Prior to Eating _____

Food and Drink Consumed/Quantities _____

_____

_____

_____

Hunger Post-Meal _____

Digestive Notes _____

_____

_____

_____

_____

Dinner

Time of Meal _____

Hunger Prior to Eating _____

Food and Drink Consumed/Quantities _____

_____

_____

_____

_____

Hunger Post-Meal _____

Digestive Notes _____

_____

_____

_____

_____

End-Of-Day Body Notes

Hours of Sleep _____

Bowel Movements _____
_____

Exercise _____
_____
_____
_____

Overall Pain _____
_____
_____
_____

DAY 9

Breakfast

Time of Meal _____

Hunger Prior to Eating_____

Food and Drink Consumed/Quantities _____

_____

_____

_____

_____

Hunger Post-Meal _____

Digestive Notes _____

_____

_____

_____

_____

Lunch

Time of Meal _____

Hunger Prior to Eating _____

Food and Drink Consumed/Quantities _____

_____

_____

_____

Hunger Post-Meal _____

Digestive Notes _____

_____

_____

_____

_____

Dinner

Time of Meal _____

Hunger Prior to Eating _____

Food and Drink Consumed/Quantities _____

_____

_____

_____

_____

Hunger Post-Meal _____

Digestive Notes _____

_____

_____

_____

_____

End-Of-Day Body Notes

Hours of Sleep _____

Bowel Movements _____

_____

Exercise _____

_____

_____

_____

Overall Pain _____

_____

_____

DAY 10

Breakfast

Time of Meal _____

Hunger Prior to Eating _____

Food and Drink Consumed/Quantities _____

_____

_____

_____

_____

Hunger Post-Meal _____

Digestive Notes _____

_____

_____

_____

_____

Lunch

Time of Meal _____

Hunger Prior to Eating _____

Food and Drink Consumed/Quantities _____

_____

_____

_____

Hunger Post-Meal _____

Digestive Notes _____

_____

_____

_____

_____

Dinner

Time of Meal _____

Hunger Prior to Eating _____

Food and Drink Consumed/Quantities _____

_____

_____

_____

_____

Hunger Post-Meal _____

Digestive Notes _____

_____

_____

_____

_____

End-Of-Day Body Notes

Hours of Sleep _____

Bowel Movements _____

_____

Exercise _____

_____

_____

_____

Overall Pain _____

_____

_____

As you complete the diets, you'll find it helpful to compare your journal entries from before the diet with those after. Highlight which foods caused problems, where you felt great, and how much improvement you felt overall. Being conscious of your body and the way it has changed is of great importance as you move into the reintroduction stage and beyond.

REMINDERS AND CLOSING NOTES FROM THE DOCTOR

Although we have come to the end of this book, your life of renewed health is just beginning. As you begin to live without the *Back Pain Relief Diet* book in hand, it's important to find the balance of both enjoying your life and feeling your best. I'll leave you with these last reminders to carry with you so that you can navigate the world of digestion with ease and comfort!

KICKSTART YOUR DAY.

Drink a large glass of cold water first thing in the morning. This should stimulate your digestive process and jump start your body's ability to eliminate your waste products. Remember, your back will only function as well as how your bowels function!

LISTEN TO YOUR BODY!

Your body speaks to you after eating. Rather than listening to what is generally known about "healthy" foods, listen to your body. How you feel and how you excrete give you the best possible information on how your digestive system is working and how optimal your diet is.

MIX IT UP!

Too much of a good thing applies even to health food! Variety is a vital part in a well-functioning digestive system. Make sure that you are avoiding your old food rut and also getting a bit of the entire food pyramid, the standard guide to healthy eating from the five basic food groups: grains, vegetables, fruits, proteins, and dairy.

EVERYTHING IN MODERATION.

This is truly the key to lifelong success. I want you to enjoy the good things in life. Diets shouldn't be restrictive. A piece of birthday cake is meant to be enjoyed. Don't overdo it, and don't deprive yourself. Both roads are detrimental to your mind and body!

I hope you have found relief from pain and a new understanding about your own body from this process. I encourage you to always treat your body as one, whole functioning system rather than a bunch of unrelated parts. I am certain that you will find truer solutions and greater back and body comfort with this in mind.

Here's to your health!

—*Dr. Todd Sinett*

THE DOCTOR'S NOTE

Digestive issues are often resolved by changing what you put in your mouth as well as what you are able to excrete. Sometimes, however, there are diseases such as Crohn's, IBS, or severe allergies that need expert attention. If you have back pain stemming from digestive issues, and you did not find relief by following the diets in this book for at least three weeks, deeper allergies or stomach problems may be at work. In that case, there are two types of experts one can consult:

- A **certified nutritionist** has in-depth knowledge and training not just in foods and diets but also in vitamins. A vitamin or mineral deficiency could be the cause of your back pain. Nutritionists can help guide you on specifically which foods to eat and which foods to avoid. They also can teach you how to analyze labels or even show you how to look at a menu and pick the proper foods when you're dining out. This can be tricky to do on your own, especially if you are someone who eats out frequently. You may have been making missteps in your diet that you weren't even aware of.

- An **internist** or **gastroenterologist** might be necessary if you have done the diet and met with a nutritionist and still feel that something isn't right with your digestive system. A specialist can examine you to make sure that there aren't any underlying issues or problems. These providers are great diagnosticians and can also prescribe the necessary medications that will not only ease your digestive function but will also help alleviate your back pain.

ACKNOWLEDGMENTS

Thanks to Jayne Pillemer, my editor, whose efforts in bringing my unique writing style into a legible form can never be appreciated enough.

To Pauline Neuwirth, my publisher, who has always been supportive and super helpful throughout the process while exhibiting some fabulous style.

To Willow Jarosh and Stephanie Clarke from CandJ Nutrition for their unparalleled knowledge of diet and nutrition.

To my wonderful staff and colleagues at Tru Whole Care, whom I have the privilege of working with every day.

To Tasman Rubel, who manages my practice and professional life with ease.

To my beloved wife for still thinking that I am funny and entertaining.

To my wonderful kids, whom I love helping with their health homework.

To my mother and sister, who are my examples of strength and perseverance since my father passed away.

Lastly, to my patients, who are my daily inspiration: they have helped me never work a day in my life.

INDEX